WITHDRAWN 19/06/24.

RESEARCH IN MEDICINE
A guide to writing a thesis in the medical sciences

RESEARCH IN MEDICINE
A guide to writing a thesis in the
medical sciences

GEORGE MURRELL, MBBS (Adelaide), DPhil (Oxon)

*Division of Orthopaedic Surgery
Duke University Medical Center,
Durham, USA*

CHRISTOPHER HUANG, PhD (Cantab), DM (Oxon)

*Physiological Laboratory,
Downing Street, Cambridge, UK*

HAROLD ELLIS, CBE, FRCS, MCh, DM (Oxon)

*Department of Anatomy,
Downing Street, Cambridge, UK*

With line drawings by
DAVID LANGDON, OBE, FRSA

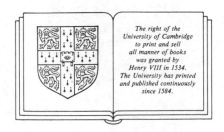

The right of the
University of Cambridge
to print and sell
all manner of books
was granted by
Henry VIII in 1534.
The University has printed
and published continuously
since 1584.

CAMBRIDGE UNIVERSITY PRESS
Cambridge
New York   Port Chester
Melbourne   Sydney

Published by the Press Syndicate of the University of Cambridge
The Pitt Building, Trumpington Street, Cambridge CB2 1RP
40 West 20th Street, New York, NY 10011, USA
10 Stamford Road, Oakleigh, Melbourne 3166, Australia

First published 1990

Printed in Great Britain by Redwood Press Ltd, Melksham, Wiltshire

British Library cataloguing in publication data
Murrell, George
Research in medicine: a guide to writing a thesis in the
medical sciences.
1. Medicine. Research
I. Title II. Huang, Christopher III. Ellis, Harold
610.72

Library of Congress cataloguing in publication data available

ISBN 0 521 39043 5 hardback
ISBN 0 521 39925 4 paperback

WD

Contents

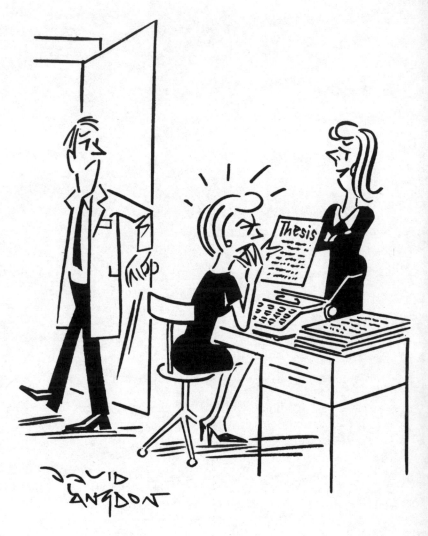

'Heavens! You don't expect intelligible writing
from doctors . . . '

Preface

Looking back on my own scientific work I should say that it shows no great originality but a certain amount of business instinct which leads to the selection of a profitable line.

E. D. Adrian, autobiographical notes [A. L. Hodgkin (1979): *Biographical Memoirs of Fellows of the Royal Society* 25, 1–73.]

Doctors and medical students experience a training directed primarily towards clinical practice. Yet, increasing numbers of the more successful additionally devote time to advancing knowl-edge, often while working for a research degree. Similarly, science students are selected for postgraduate work mainly through university degree results. However, little is said about the qualities one requires for successfully completing a research programme, and the extent to which these differ from what makes a successful doctor or undergraduate student. No doubt one requires originality, creativity or flair, but to attempt to define or expand upon these would be beyond the direct scope of this short book. Additionally, modern medicine encompasses an enormous breadth of subjects, and research is among the most individual of endeavours.

Nevertheless, one can discuss some of the more practical problems associated with pursuing research and working for a thesis. We do feel that a capacity to tackle these fulfils a necessary, even if not a sufficient, condition for a successful postgraduate programme. We hope we have commented helpfully upon at least some of these hurdles, even if only briefly in a general way. If we thereby provoke constructive thought, even if not agreement, we shall feel we have achieved our object and have offered assistance to those seeking masterships, doctorates and honours degrees.

We are most grateful to Mrs Teresa Smith for so patiently converting our frequently unintelligible writings into manuscript; the Universities of Cambridge and London for providing us with their degree regulations; Dr Richard Barling of Cambridge University Press; and Professor R. H. Adrian of the Physiological Laboratory, University of Cambridge for guidance and encouragement. Finally, having much enjoyed David Langdon's cartoons in *Punch*, we particularly appreciate his humorous and sensitive illustrations of what might otherwise have been rather over-serious material.

George Murrell
Chris Huang
Harold Ellis

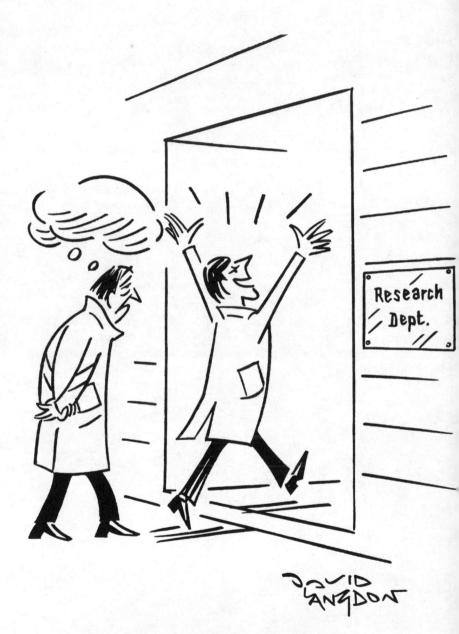

Frustrating . . . or rewarding . . .

1

Introduction

Aims of this book

This guide was written primarily for medical students and practitioners considering whether to attempt a programme involving original research in the medical and biological sciences. The author who initiated this text (GM) read for a medical degree, did a stint in research and has now returned to clinical medicine with an academic interest. He was then joined by two others, one of whom (CH) first qualified in medicine and has subsequently remained in research, and another (HE) who has had a primarily academic medical career. Accordingly, the authors themselves represent the major groups of people who do medical research.

Individuals have different reasons for wishing to do research, which include gaining a higher degree. Such a pursuit can be incredibly exhilarating and rewarding. Alternatively, it can be an endless, lonely, boring and frustrating exercise. The aim of this monograph is to guide the potential medical postgraduate candidate away from the latter predicament. It is not intended to dictate the researcher's own originality, creativity or scientific approach. Rather, it is organized around a sequence of practical steps directed at the more pragmatic questions:

'What steps do I take?'
'When and where do I start?'
'How do I get to the end of the tunnel?'
'What do I do next?'

1

We thereby hope to alleviate unnecessary anxiety and save the reader valuable time and energy that could then be used in a more productive way. We have accordingly set out much of the text in a simple, didactic format.

Much of what we outline will be simple common sense, but we hope that our presentation will enable the reader to pick out 'the wood from the trees' and assist the reader to his or her task with greater efficiency and confidence. Our comments are directed largely at academic doctors. However, the basic principles of maintaining an effective individual research programme can be applied to all experimental sciences.

Time frame

This guide is organized in the chronological order of the steps most doctors take when pursuing a research programme. Everyone first has to decide whether he or she wishes to pursue research. This is considered in the next chapter. If a research programme is chosen, it can be for different lengths of time, varying from a few months to a lifetime. Nevertheless research programmes tend to fall into four phases. Following the necessary background preparation in the area to be studied, one establishes and develops methods to be used in the research project ('setting up phase'). Time is then needed to assess the limitations of these methods and to develop one's experimental skills to a level where they yield valid results ('frustration phase'). There then follows serious hypothesis testing and obtaining and analysing results ('results phase'). Finally the results are written up and communicated ('writing up phase'). The time and emphasis bearing on each of these steps varies with person and project. In particular, the prominence of the 'frustration phase' varies greatly with circumstances and the good or ill fortune of the investigator. We shall devote most attention to the first and last phases for which even a wide variety of research programmes will have much in common. The time taken to write up the thesis usually increases exponentially with the total time set aside by the doctor for research.

The following table gives a typical expectation of the relative lengths of these hypothetical phases, for different durations of research project. The latter is discussed further in Chapter 3. In order to be realistic, a brief period of holiday is allowed for in each scheme:

Completion time	Setting up	Frustration	Results	Writing up	Holiday
1 year	4 weeks	4 weeks	30 weeks	10 weeks	4 weeks
2 years	3 months	3 months	10 months	6 months	2 months
3 years	3 months	8 months	11 months	11 months	3 months

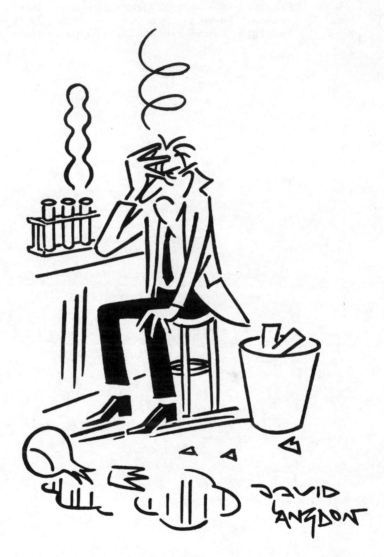

Great potential for disasters . . .

2

Why do research?

Research experience is increasingly important in today's fight for jobs and so the aspiring clinician may leap, somewhat reluctantly, into a research programme without carefully assessing its processes, outcomes, advantages and disadvantages. Some considerations as to whether one should do research at all are presented here.

The challenge

Research by its very nature offers a tremendous intellectual and personal challenge and additionally has the potential to unearth information that may help the wider community.

Becoming a better clinician

It can be argued that many of the qualities necessary for, and consequently developed in, research (an open, inquiring mind, logical thought, careful analysis of previous research with a mild degree of scepticism, an understanding of the processes necessary to achieve the presented result, self discipline and self sufficiency), are also of considerable value in clinical practice. Almost any established clinicians who have spent time in research during their training, whether they are surgeons in district general hospitals, physicians in private practice or general practitioners, will tell you that they regard themselves better doctors as a result of this experience. They find themselves more able to analyse a clinical problem, appraise the results of their management of patients and assess objectively the latest claims from scientists, colleagues and pharmaceutical companies because of their exposure to the scientific method.

As part of an academic career

Without doubt, research achievement, including a higher degree by thesis, is essential for a career in academic medicine. Most people who decide on a career in university medicine do so from an interest in research and teaching; it is not invariably true but it is surprising how often the two do go together! It is a hard fact that subsequent promotion in such a career depends heavily on a proven research record with relevant publications in reputable and refereed journals.

Competing in the job market

Selecting one applicant rather than another in appointments for medical jobs is a difficult process. One way to help differentiate candidates, which appears to be becoming increasingly popular, is to consider their ability to conduct research and their having research publications. Several good papers in reputable journals consequently serve a candidate well for future (particularly academically inclined) employment. However, one must remember that two or three years in an unproductive pursuit of research away from any clinical experience, leading to a few esoteric papers, may not enhance your status with some future employers, particularly if they have no special interest in research.

Fame

Potential for fame on a small scale is good. You could well find yourself making significant new discoveries, getting a difficult assay to work or solving a theoretical problem. However, to reach great heights actually requires years of dedication, insight and luck. On the other hand, there is a great potential for disasters (unsuccessful projects, infected cultures, broken glassware and machinery, etc.) and wasting months or years in the pursuit of what seems to be an endless unsolvable problem.

Lifestyle

If you want continual reassurance and direction, research is not for you. Self assurance, independent thought, and the willingness to take a chance are valuable in research. The working day is structured by you, not your employer, but this does leave greater freedom for other activities. The distinction between work and rest is less clear and there is great pressure on you to work at home and on weekends. Monetary rewards while in research are generally less than in clinical medicine.

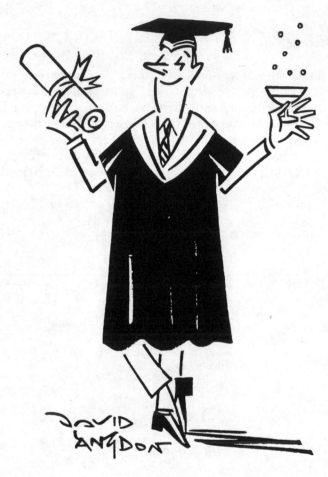

Higher degree . . .

3

Reading for a research degree

Most doctors doing a period of research will wish to work for a higher university degree. The degree one attempts depends on a number of factors. These include:

- what you can realistically achieve,
- the time required for completion,
- your own qualifications,
- individual university regulations,
- funding available,
- the subject matter you wish to study,
- the country where you wish to work.

What degrees are available?

Some United Kingdom and Commonwealth universities encourage their medical (undergraduate) students to enter for intercalated Bachelor of Medical Science (BMedSc) or Bachelor of Science (BSc) degrees. Others offer postgraduate Master of Philosophy (MPhil) or Master of Science (MSc) degrees. In the United States, the MD (Doctorate of Medicine) is the basic medical degree, not a higher research-based medical degree, as in the United Kingdom and Commonwealth. Most universities offer a Doctorate of Philosophy (PhD or DPhil). Some United States universities (as will the Universities of Oxford and Cambridge, UK) have a combined MD/PhD programme. Most universities in the United Kingdom and Common-wealth also award an MS (Master of Surgery) degree for surgical candidates, which is equivalent to the MD for medical candidates by thesis. Other universities have abandoned the MS and, at these universities, the surgical candidates submit an MD thesis alongside their medical colleagues, and are subject to the same regulations. The standard (and often the regulations) for the degree of MS and MD are considered equivalent.

Local regulations must be studied carefully. For example, the Master of Surgery of the University of Cambridge requires the candidate to pass a tough examination (which comprises essay papers, clinical and oral examinations), *after* his or her thesis has been approved.

Time required for completion

You will certainly have views about the length of time you wish to devote to research, and this will influence what you attempt. A doctorate is the most substantial qualification but takes a longer time. Examples of completion times for postgraduate degrees include:

Bachelor of Medical Science (BMedSc)	1 year
Intercalated Bachelor of Science (BSc)	1 year
Master of Philosophy (MPhil)	1–2 years
Master of Science (MSc)	1–2 years
Doctor of Philosophy (PhD or DPhil)	2–4 years
Doctor of Medicine (MD or DM)	2–3 years
Master of Surgery (MS or MCh)	2–3 years

Your own qualifications

Entry to a higher degree requires acceptance by both the university and the department in which you wish to work. The level of degree for which your application would be eligible will vary with your own academic background. In the United Kingdom, studentships, scholarships and fellowships for which you may apply for financial support often require an honours degree with a II.1 or higher final grade. In addition, you need to check particular regulations very carefully: many universities only allow their own graduates to attempt their higher degrees, particularly medical doctorates. Other universities allow external applications.

Individual university regulations

Different universities vary widely in their regulations and requirements even for equivalent higher degrees. It is therefore important to check such details with the admissions office or the postgraduate dean of your prospective university, particularly if it is not your undergraduate university. You should also study carefully the postgraduate prospectuses, to get an idea of available departments, and the research areas they offer. The scope and quality of postgraduate research varies greatly between universities, and even between departments in the same university. Finally, it is prudent to seek advice from someone recently embarked on the programme you are considering, once you become interested in a particular department.

Doctor of Medicine (MD or DM)

Clinical candidates typically opt for the Doctor of Medicine. To be eligible, candidates are generally required to have held a primary medical degree of the university concerned for a minimum of typically five years and to be fully registered with the General Medical Council. The stringency of additional requirements varies with university. For example, London University requires candidates to hold its own Bachelor of Medicine & Bachelor of Surgery (MBBS). Cambridge University simply requires candidates to hold one of its primary degrees (this includes the BA), and a registrable medical qualification. A typical MD thesis deals with a topic in medicine, or any branch of medicine, or medical science. It typically embodies original findings, and observes certain conditions of presentation and overall length. In addition, candidates are frequently examined *viva voce*. If clinical research is involved, full ethical approval must have been obtained.

Most universities advise their candidates to seek more senior advice in the field covered by the proposed thesis at an early stage. Some universities exceptionally allow a submission in the form of previously published work rather than a thesis.

Master of Surgery (MS)

The Master of Surgery is more popular with surgical candidates, although some now opt for the MD. Again, typically, the candidate must have held a medical degree for not less than five years, and have spent not less than two years in training posts in surgery or in a special branch of surgery approved by one of the Royal Colleges of Surgery, and be fully registered with the General Medical Council. London University requires candidates to hold its own Bachelor of Medicine & Bachelor of Surgery, but Cambridge simply requires a primary degree and a registrable medical qualification. The thesis would deal with a topic in general surgery or with some special branch of surgery, and there may also be an oral examination.

Doctor of Philosophy (PhD or DPhil)

Regulations for PhD degrees are even more varied. These usually entail residence and full-time research in the university over stipulated times (two to three years; not less than three years in the University of Cambridge). This degree cannot normally be attempted while simultaneously holding a primarily clinical attachment. However, registration for a PhD usually only requires a first degree and does not require full clinical qualifications as demanded by MD or MS regulations. Thus, one can begin work for a PhD immediately after one's primary medical qualification or intercalated BSc.

Shorter degree courses (MSc, MPhil, etc.) usually also stipulate a period of full-time work resident in the university but also can be taken very soon after one's primary qualification.

Available funding

Most universities charge fees when one is working in residence for a higher academic degree. If you have a grant or scholarship to cover such expenses, consider attempting the longer, more prestigious degree. If you are self funded, a shorter, less expensive higher medical degree may be more practicable. Medical Research Council fellowships may be available, usually funded at a senior house officer level (without payments for providing medical cover outside normal hours), to work for research degrees. Grants and scholarships offer considerably lower stipends than do full-time clinical appointments and so periods in full-time research entail significant financial sacrifice. In addition, a considerable fee component is payable in the case of MSc, MPhil and PhD degrees. However the time when one can attempt a PhD or MSc in relation to one's qualification date is flexible. In the UK and Commonwealth, the MD and MS are usually taken as career degrees and so recurrent fees are usually not charged. In addition, apart from a requirement for full medical qualification, the regulations regarding completion time, subject and supervisor for these latter two higher degrees are less tight.

If, at the outset, you decide upon a one year MSc course, bear in mind that it may not be possible to 'upgrade' this to a PhD should you wish to do so in the course of the work, and the year you are supported may still be deducted from subsequent research support by some funding councils.

Prestige

A PhD is considered by some to carry most scientific weight. Some medical circles may regard an MD or MS as more relevant, especially for a future career in a branch of clinical medicine or surgery.

Subject matter

There are usually relatively few restrictions concerning exact subject matter for higher degrees, but each university has its own particular regulations. A PhD, MSc or BMedSc is often orientated more towards basic sciences, while an MD or MS is more clinically biased in subject matter. However, overlap can and does occur and so many MD or MS theses are entirely laboratory based, although one would expect these latter to have some clinical relevance.

Providing for your future career

Anyone planning a medical career will naturally wonder about the consequences of 'time out' for research and whether this would have any possible adverse effects on future prospects.

A year or two of research taken out of an undergraduate career leading to a BSc, MPhil or PhD, is a well-recognized step in most universities. Indeed, this is often actively encouraged for the more successful and presents no academic problems for re-entry into a medical course. The only disadvantage is that you lose a number of your friends in your year, whom you find when you return to the mainstream clinical teaching are now a year or two ahead of you – but, after all, you now have an extra degree!

The decision to do research off-service during your postgraduate medical training certainly requires careful consideration of how you are going to re-enter your clinical programme. Ideally, you could take a post which includes a year or more off-service specifically for research as a part of a planned rotation. These unfortunately seem to be becoming less common in the United Kingdom owing to progressive government economies. Other appointments to research posts may be accompanied by an assurance from your employers that they will do their very best to get you back into the clinical training programme at their institution. This is more likely to be achieved successfully when the appointment is in the laboratories of a large university hospital, especially if it has affiliations or rotation schemes with a number of district hospitals.

Less happy is the situation when you deliberately take a research post without anything definite to go to when this comes to an end. Under these circumstances, you must bear in mind the importance of seeking a future position in good time – otherwise you may find yourself in the dole queue!

One thing that gives some encouragement is that many training programmes (the Surgical Senior Registrar Scheme in the United Kingdom, for example) will recognize a year of full-time research towards their requirements, and you should check this early on when you are planning to go 'off-service'.

Medical careers in different English-speaking countries

Most of this book concerns individuals in the United Kingdom, but it may be helpful to compare the nature of medical careers in the United States and Australia, as the variations mean that a research stint will have different implications for one's medical career. The remarks in each of the next three sections are organized as follows:

1. The basic undergraduate degree
2. Research degrees
3. Postgraduate medical training
4. Post-specialist training

Under each category we shall consider the following:

- time taken
- structure of the training programme, if any
- nature of examinations or assessment
- costs or remuneration

There are major differences between systems in these three countries; indeed each country throughout the world has evolved its own peculiar rules and regulations. However, probably every graduate (and indeed most undergraduates) will be familiar with the situation in his or her own country. The important point is that if you propose to do part of your training (and particularly your research) in a foreign country, it behoves you to find out as much as you can about the career programme both in your host country and university well before you arrive there.

There is of course no reason why you should not do your laboratory or clinical research overseas and submit the material as an MD or MS thesis to your own university.

United Kingdom

(1) The undergraduate medical course typically lasts five years from leaving school at 18. Entry is highly competitive, and based on school academic performance. It usually consists of a two year course in basic medical sciences and three years of exposure to a wide range of clinical subjects before obtaining the primary medical qualification to practise. Candidates at Oxford, Cambridge and a number of other medical schools do a third preclinical year leading to an honours degree. Other universities offer the opportunity of an intercalated BSc to selected candidates. The medical course is highly structured with rigorous assessment of both theoretical and practical work every 3–12 months. Educational costs are currently government-funded for resident United Kingdom nationals. Overseas students outside the European Economic Community pay full economic cost fees.

(2) The scientific research degree is typically the Doctor of Philos-

ophy (PhD or DPhil) taking 2–4 years to complete. It is almost entirely a research degree with little or no formal course work. Assessment is through thesis and oral examination, usually conducted by an internal and external examiner. United Kingdom nationals can receive financial support through research council grants but overseas nationals pay fees.

The clinical scientific research degrees are the Doctor of Medicine (MD or DM) and Master of Surgery (MS or MChir); note that in the United States the MD is the basic medical degree rather than such a senior qualification. Award of the MD is through research, like the PhD. Award of the MS may require a clinical examination. These degrees can often be worked for while holding other clinical appointments for flexible periods of time. This is in contrast to a formal residence requirement in full-time research required by the PhD.

(3) Postgraduate medical training in the United Kingdom varies with speciality. Typically it includes:

i. a one year internship (pre-registration positions) consisting of six months supervised work respectively in medicine and surgery;
ii. at least two years of senior house officer posts, each lasting around six months, but which could be organized into a rotation;
iii. at least two years of registrar positions;
iv. at least three years of a senior registrar position before application for consultant vacancies.

Unfortunately, at present, phases (ii) and (iii) are usually considerably longer, particularly in general medicine or surgery.

Formal assessment varies with speciality but generally involves:

i. a primary Membership (in medicine, and obstetrics and gynaecology) or Fellowship (in surgery or pathology) examination organized by the Royal College in the speciality, evaluating the candidate's command of basic principles, including basic sciences, at between one and three years after full registration.
ii. part 2 of a Membership (medicine, and obstetrics and gynaecology) or Fellowship (in surgery or pathology) examination around four years after qualification with a more clinical emphasis.

There are currently discussions concerning the introduction of further 'exit' examinations in particular specialities: these are about to be initiated by the Surgical Royal Colleges.* These examinations are

*The regulations for the primary and final examinations for the Fellowship of the Royal College of Surgeons (FRCS) are due for some quite radical changes

taken while candidates are in service in recognized training positions, which vary in the amount of formal instruction being offered.

(4) Post-specialist training occurs along two major streams in the United Kingdom.

i. There are academic grades of clinical lecturer, university lecturer and senior lecturers, reader and professor, where a substantial proportion of one's stipend originates from the university system, and where there is frequently a substantial research commitment.
ii. There are more directly vocational consultant positions in the National Health Service.

Australia

(1) and (2) The arrangements for first degree (MBBS), PhD, MD and MS qualification and post-specialist training are similar to those in the United Kingdom.

(3) Arrangements for postgraduate medical training differ somewhat from those in the United Kingdom.

i. There is a one year internship but with often shorter rotations through more medical and surgical specialities.
ii. This is followed by two years of general specialist training with rotations every three months through subspecialities.
iii. There may then be one to two years of work in service positions.
iv. Finally, there is a four year specialist training programme, also rotating every three months.

Postgraduate medical training is therefore well structured, with fresh job applications only required at two levels.

(4) Postgraduate examinations also differ slightly. There are primary Membership or Fellowship examinations in basic sciences at 1–3 years after one's primary medical qualifications. However, Part 2 Membership or Fellowship examinations tend to mark the end of speciality training, and are directed to cover the specific specialities.

United States of America

(1) The basic medical degree is the MD. Candidates undergo a four year 'premedical' undergraduate course which allows a liberal

but, at the time of going to press, these have not yet been published. Candidates should contact the Secretary of their appropriate College for details of the new examinations.

choice of subjects. They then compete for places in a highly structured four year medical course. These are heavily examined, often by
multiple choice examinations. In addition, some individual states
impose medical qualifying examinations before allowing a medical
graduate to practise in that state. Fees are payable and vary widely
between universities.

(2) There is only one major research doctorate at most universities,
the PhD, which takes four to five years. PhD programmes in the
United States are highly structured in the first two years, with laboratory and course work. Some universities offer a medical Master of
Science (MS or MSc) which is a one year research programme with
thesis.

Some US universities set written qualifying examinations at the
end of the second year of a PhD programme. They may also require
a *viva voce* examination on the research proposal. Frequently, there
are intra-departmental committees to monitor research progress,
with reviews every six months. Final examination includes submission of a thesis.

(3) Postgraduate medical training in the United States lasts four to
six years (including the internship). It is highly structured with organized rotations through medical or surgical specialities during the first
two years, followed by rotation through the chosen speciality, with
the candidates progressively assuming greater clinical responsibility
during the training period. Assessment is informal during training,
often through self assessment multiple choice tests. However, formal
'Speciality Board' examinations take place at the end of the training
programme.

(4) The emphasis of post-specialist training can be either primarily
academic or primarily vocational.

i. Short-term academic 'fellowships' can be taken in particular
   subspecialities. There is then a hierarchy, including assistant, associate,
   and full professor. Assessment at this stage is by faculty or by peer review.
ii. Vocational positions in the private sector are very flexible. Assessments
    are being introduced ('grandfather' examinations) for those long in prac-
    tice.

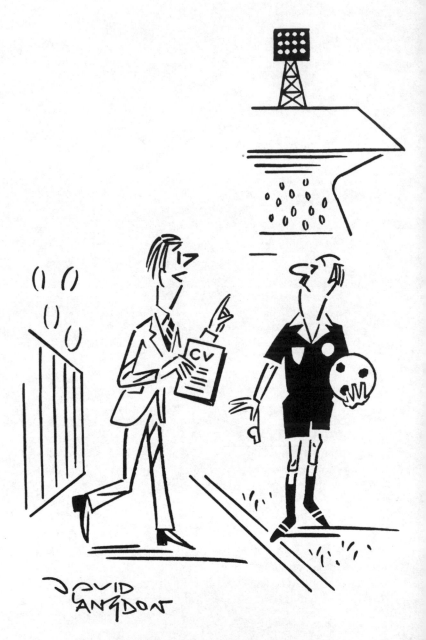

Approaching referees . . .

4

Applying for research positions

Having decided to pursue a research project, and upon the qualification you wish to attempt, you next need to apply for a suitable position. This chapter will consider this exercise in the following order:

- Timing your period of research
- Choice of department
- Applying for scholarships and research positions
- Background information about the available position
- Your curriculum vitae
- Approaching referees

Timing your period of research

Biological scientists not proceeding to do medicine usually attempt their higher degrees immediately after their first degree, often continuing an interest arising from an honours degree project. Others return to university, after a time working in industry. Medical students or doctors have three major options.

Research before the undergraduate clinical course

A number of medical students become sufficiently interested in basic sciences, and consequently in postgraduate work, before their three year clinical undergraduate course. This is particularly so if they have read for an honours degree, or included an intercalated BSc. Under such circumstances, you have the advantage of having basic scientific concepts fresh in your mind and this can be helpful at least at the beginning. Doing your research at this stage also avoids disruption to clinical training later.

However, your research would then be confined to experimental scientific work. You would have neither the knowledge of, nor the access to, a clinical environment except under very particular circumstances determined by the interests and background of your supervisor. It is not possible to be a candidate for an MS or MD before fully qualifying in medicine. You will also have to complete your work within a strict time limit in order to rejoin your medical course, at the appropriate point in the academic year. Clinical schools are often helpful and understanding when allowing clinical places to be deferred to allow a student to attempt an advanced research degree. However, the deferral is necessarily for a fixed time, limited by the start of the academic year.

Research after full clinical registration

An alternative is to enter a period of research immediately after completing your internship (pre-registration) year. This takes you three to four years away from your undergraduate basic science. On the other hand, you will have acquired some clinical experience, and won some time to decide upon your interests. This is more helpful than you think: it is difficult to have the perspective to decide on important research areas during or immediately after a first degree course. A full medical qualification also enhances your access to clinical projects, although you will not yet have the specialist medical knowledge which comes from working for postgraduate medical examinations. You must also bear in mind that you will have left clinical medicine at a relatively junior stage in your career, and so will have to arrange to re-enter at the bottom of the medical hierarchy after your 'time out'.

Research during clinical specialist training

An increasing number of hospital doctors incorporate a period of research into their postgraduate (specialist) training. This has the advantage that you will have the specialist clinical knowledge to select areas that you regard as being interesting and important. You may be rather more out of touch with the basic medical sciences, but some serious reading will soon remedy this gap. However, a research stint seems a more noticeable interruption of career at this stage and one then also has to consider financial implications and family commitments.

Research preceding the internship year

A fourth option, which we would not recommend, is to do research between the primary medical degree and pre-registration clinical attachments. This option almost completely prevents a subsequent career in clinical medicine. A year as a pre-registration house officer or an intern is a prerequisite in all countries for practising medicine. To go back to this after time in research is logistically and psychologically difficult. In addition, it is during your internship that you acquire much of your knowledge of medical practice, and this could be very beneficial to your subsequent medical research.

Choice of department

After deciding on the timing for your research programme, you next need to decide where you would like to conduct your research and how you will fund it. Applications for funding support almost always require you to state the field in which you plan to do your research and, in general terms, what you wish to do. Once successful in gaining support, you are expected to follow your plans through, although you may be permitted to make minor adjustments to arrangements more suitable for your needs.

One place to start is a university or clinical department whose work or interest lies close to interests in your desired career path. For instance, if you would like ultimately to be a transplant surgeon, you might try the local university department of surgery. Alternatively you may wish to work with a specific individual whose work you are familiar with and regard highly. If your career plans have not yet crystallized, the decision is more difficult. At all events, it is prudent to learn a little about any particular department you are considering. You should consider trying the following:

1. A computer search (see Chapter 6) to find the range and scope of publications produced over recent years by that department.
2. Consulting previous students who have worked in that department. This is invaluable. It could provide you with detailed information about the areas being studied, and about the scientists who work there.
3. Consulting a more senior colleague, who is now in the kind of position you would like eventually to achieve yourself, about the academic and research standing of that department.

Applying for scholarships and research positions

Having decided on a particular department or research unit, and having confirmed that it offers research opportunities, either through a postgraduate programme or advertisements of research positions, you may consider making an application. This entails, in not necessarily chronological order, as this would vary with circumstances:

1. selecting an area to study;
2. weighing up the facilities available in that department for your study (see Chapter 5);
3. obtaining background information about the department or position;
4. setting out information about yourself;
5. finding referees who will write about you;
6. selecting a supervisor (see Chapter 5);
7. applying for financial support.

Having assembled your application you must ensure it arrives at the appropriate place in time for the closing date. One would normally send one's documentation by recorded post or by hand. Other means of communication if you are pressed by a time limit include:

FAX: a FAX machine is a combination of a telex and a photocopier. You dial the number of the receiving FAX machine and then feed your documents (for example, your letter of application and curriculum vitae) through the machine as you would a photocopier. The machine at the other end receives them in a matter of seconds and sends back an acknowledgement. The cost is equivalent to a telephone call for the time it takes to transmit the documents.

E-Mail: this is a computer-linked system, particularly popular in the United States, by which users of mainframe computers can search and apply for jobs. To apply for a job, the user simply sends his letter of application, and curriculum vitae (which is already on the computer) through the electronic mail. A very fast and convenient service.

Background information about the available position

Find out, usually from the departmental secretary or postgraduate tutor, the selection procedure. In particular you might like to know:

1. who is on the selection committee;
2. the closing date for applications;
3. how many candidates will be short listed;
4. the date, place, time and length of interview;
5. how many candidates will be selected and how many posts are available;
6. when the decision will be announced.

Visit your future place of employment, particularly when deciding upon a research supervisor or if you are already interested in one. Many departments will prefer candidates who have already approached, and been regarded as acceptable for, research supervision by a particular staff member. Talk with those who have been or who are already there, ask about the work conducted there, possible supervisors, etc.

Your curriculum vitae

You next need to furnish information about yourself to your possible future employers. A curriculum vitae is almost always required for any job or scholarship application. It is the major means by which you convey details of yourself in postgraduate applications and may be the only thing your potential employers see before drawing up a short list for the interview. It is accordingly imperative to give the best account of yourself. Make sure your curriculum vitae is typed out clearly and neatly with a good-quality printer. It is useful to store your curriculum vitae on a word processor, so that you can add to and modify it as your career progresses.

The following particulars must be included in a curriculum vitae:

1. Name
2. Address

3. Date of birth
4. Nationality
5. Current and previous positions held
6. School education
7. University education
8. Qualifications with dates
9. Scholarships, prizes and academic awards
10. Positions of responsibility in chronological order
11. Membership of professional organizations
12. Publications
13. Interests and hobbies
14. Names and addresses of referees

Approaching referees

Most job applications require you to supply names (and addresses) of two or three referees. They should preferably be:

1. previous employers or teachers who know you and your work well;
2. themselves in fields relevant to your application;
3. people whom you believe to have a good opinion of your own work and academic performance.

Once you have decided which referees you want:

1. write to them asking if they would mind supporting your application;
2. send them a copy of your application and a summary of what you have done since they were last in contact with you;
3. give them a brief account of the position for which you are applying;
4. let them know the eventual outcome of your application, thanking them, particularly if you are successful.

Graduate work in the United States

Graduate programmes in the United States are considerably more organized than in the United Kingdom with explicitly advertised courses and periods of research. It is often therefore necessary to apply in a more formal way, usually on forms with instructions obtained from the dean of the graduate school. Applications usually have to be accompanied by an 'academic transcript' and confidential letters of evaluation, sent directly to the graduate school. Depending on the admitting departments, American candidates often additionally take Graduate Record Examination (GRE) general and subject tests. It is likely that a foreign candidate, particularly a British hon-ours degree holder, may have such requirements modified. How-ever, other foreign students, particularly those from non-English speaking countries, may have to satisfy further language require-ments. This typically involves a certification of English proficiency from the Test of English as a Foreign Language (TOEFL). You may also have to produce statements confirming your financial ability to support a course of graduate study.

Owing to the more formal nature of American graduate courses, it is essential that all information is sent to the university graduate school office well before the specified deadlines. Preliminary enquiries, particularly in heavily subscribed universities, may have to begin even two years before the projected starting date.

American students often pursue graduate work on a part-time basis. However, this is not permitted for overseas students by visa regulations.

Overseas graduate students face a number of additional expenses in the United States, with which the United Kingdom graduate, for example, may not be familiar. A full-time graduate student pays a university fee every semester though this is reduced for individuals simultaneously working as teaching or research assistants. Cover must also be arranged for accident and sickness insurance. Your financial support must also cover registration, student health fees and apartment rents, in addition to meals, books and other personal expenses.

Some financial assistance is available even within US universities as fellowships and scholarships, but US Federal programmes tend to support US citizens and permanent residents only. Individual depart-ments may offer paid graduate and research assistantships.

US research degrees entail substantial course work, and satisfac-tory performance at associated examinations, and therefore differ substantially from British graduate curricula. For example, Duke University requires completion of specialist courses, a period of resi-dence, a preliminary examination, work for a dissertation and a final examination for the award of a PhD.

Information on times and places of graduate record examinations may be obtained from:

Educational Testing Service,
PO Box 6000,
Princeton, NJ 08541-6000, USA

Information on Test of English as a Foreign Language (TOEFL) may be obtained from:

Educational Testing Service,
PO Box 6155,
Princeton, NJ 08541-6155, USA

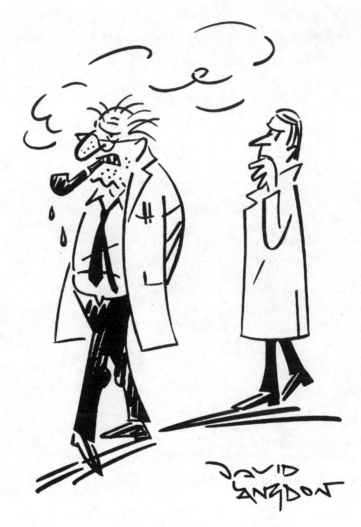

Your supervisor . . .

5

Research supervisors and projects

Even before you actually start applying for research positions, you inevitably will be thinking about the area of research you might pursue, and the person with whom you may wish to work. If you have strong ideas about these from the outset, they will determine the channels along which you will make enquiries and applications. Alternatively you may seek openings or scholarships at particular departments with initially less specific interests in mind, and seek a direction for your research afterwards. Most applicants will discover a middle course, being initially drawn towards a department, then gradually acquiring knowledge of available research areas and personnel as enquiries and the application proceed. However, whichever sequence of events you fall into, you will need to think about the following.

1. Deciding upon a research supervisor: the major personal contact that will bear upon your research.
2. Choosing a research topic: what you will work on during your period of research.
3. Considering the physical facilities and expertise accessible to you in your particular laboratory.

Your research supervisor

Your supervisor is the senior member in the laboratory to whom you will be assigned, and who will provide guidance in the course of your

31

research project. He or she will be the most important individual to your academic well-being during your time in research. He or she is likely to be someone who has research experience and who can provide the assistance and advice you need to make progress. Basically these should include:

1. a laboratory with the equipment and materials you will need;
2. initial ideas;
3. general research knowledge;
4. knowledge specific to the topic you will be investigating;
5. technical expertise;
6. a proof reader as your written work starts to appear;
7. a 'clock': your supervisor should give you indications of your progress, and encourage you to present your work to specific meetings at the appropriate time;
8. an introduction to other researchers with knowledge beyond his own should this prove necessary;
9. an introduction to future employers.

The process is not all one way. In return, your supervisor is likely to receive:

1. inexpensive research labour;
2. your own knowledge, both original and acquired;
3. your ideas, ingenuity, energy and time;
4. an expansion of his net research activity, with a possibility of publications in collaboration with you, depending on how closely you work with him.

Who should be your supervisor? There are three ways to obtain a supervisor.

1. The prospective supervisor approaches you.
2. You approach the supervisor.
3. The head of the department assigns you to a particular supervisor.

The choice of supervisor is, perhaps, the most important and most difficult of your decisions. There is a good deal of luck involved in terms of the fit of personalities and ideas. If you do not like the look of your potential supervisor, it is best to decide upon a change of supervisor at an early stage, rather than offending him or her and many others later. Perhaps to be initially non-committal is an advantage.

If you have a say in the matter, the departmental head or secretary can provide a list of academics within the department. Again it is useful to check on their publications and to talk to their previous research students. This will give you an idea of a particular supervisor's fields of interest, the size of his or her research group and the degree of contact he or she offers within the laboratory. If possible, contact or write to prospective supervisors to arrange meetings and to see their laboratory. This meeting will form a useful means of mutual assessment.

Choosing a research topic

The topic in which you choose to work for your thesis will depend on a number of factors, which include:

- your own interests and aspirations,
- your supervisor's interests,
- facilities available in the department,
- whether you wish to work on experimental or human systems.

Considering your own interests and aspirations

Clearly, if you wish to become a neurosurgeon, you will be more interested in examining 'the effects of nerve growth factor in the sensory cortex' than the 'morphogenesis of bone cells'. However, it is not always possible to get very close to your true interest. This is usually due to limitations of physical, technical or academic expertise. In these cases, you need to weigh up the advantages of expertise with its greater guarantee of success and the potentially more exciting but dangerous individualism.

Your supervisor's interests

It is likely that you will have something in mind regarding your research project. Your supervisor will also have a project in mind. The two will not always coincide. In general, it is advisable initially to follow your supervisor's ideas. He is more likely to have the research knowledge to make more informed, realistic decisions. As your work and reading progress, you will acquire the knowledge and skills to become more independent. Most supervisors will encourage this independence at the appropriate time.

The relationship between research supervisor and student is very much like a parent/child one. Most initial decisions and over-all care, including funding and housing, are provided by the parent. As the child matures, he is able to make more of his own decisions and please his parents with signs of independence. Nevertheless, the parental figure should always be there to 'rescue' the child in times of unforeseen hardship. Conversely, the child will be more productive and less obstreperous if given the freedom (at the correct time) to pursue his own interests. The relationship may then become synergistic, in which both parties learn and gain from the relationship. The parent/child analogy follows through many aspects of the supervisor/supervisee relationship, including an occasional lack of objectivity on the part of both the student and the supervisor!

Considering the laboratory facilities available

However good your reason for wishing to pursue a particular area, this will be frustrated if your laboratory does not have the requisite facilities, background or personnel. Your thesis topic will consequently be affected by a number of practical limi-tations. These include:

(1) *Laboratory workshop facilities.* A limited number of these (whether providing mechanical, electrical engineering or tissue culture support) will be available and well established in your lab-oratory. It is prudent to work on a project whose demands will be realistic in relation to what your supporting department techni-cians are accustomed to, as you will then have a source of help when in difficulty.

(2) *Expertise available.* Quite clearly, it would be most prudent to work on areas where your supervisor and his colleagues have experience and expertise. At all events, major departures from this norm must not be undertaken lightly and are risky for the inexperienced scientist.

(3) *Time available.* It is unrealistic to expect to develop a sub-stantial new technique in a limited time. In contrast, someone holding a longer-term position may try projects in areas in which the laboratory may not have experience.

(4) *Cost and funding.* In general, it is more practical and

efficient to confine your experiments to those for which your laboratory is already equipped. Frequently, your supervisor will have taken you on a grant with fairly specific provisions and terms of reference that may not readily allow for major departures in direction.

(5) *Your own expertise.* Under certain circumstances, you may have already acquired expertise in a particular technique elsewhere. You might then consider trying such a technique even if this is novel to your present laboratory. However, you must bear in mind that setting up new procedures may be unexpectedly time consuming in a different environment and this extra time must justify itself in terms of interest or results.

(6) *Subjects.* You will need something or someone upon which to conduct your research. In general terms, medical research can be conducted on (1) cells and tissues, (2) animals or (3) humans. Different departments or laboratories will have different capacities in these areas. Each system has its own advantages and disadvantages; some of these are briefly commented on below.

Human medical research

Research involving humans is often thought to be the most obviously applicable to clinical medicine. There are several approaches to studying human populations. These include the following:

(1) *Observation or intervention.* You may simply observe particular phenomena in your human subjects, for example, the proportion of patients with a palmaris longus tendon in a population of patients with and without Dupuytren's contracture. Alternatively, you may conduct a clinical trial, where one form of intervention or management is assessed against another, for example, the effect of total mastectomy with or without radiotherapy on the five-year survival of patients with breast cancer.

(2) *Population studies.* A study may describe a single case of a given condition or treatment (e.g. the first splenic transplant), a sample of a given population, or the whole population (e.g. the incidence of skin cancer in Faeroe Islanders).

(3) *Prospective or retrospective trials.* A prospective study makes an initial assessment on a given population and then fol-

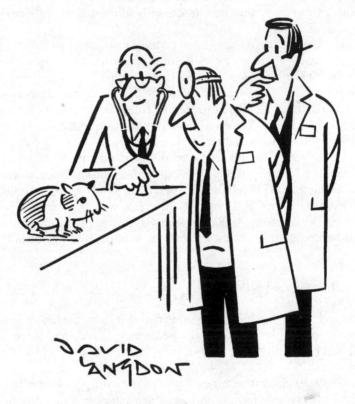

Less clinically applicable . . .

lows up the same group over a period of time. A retrospective study looks backwards in time, after the event, for example, looking up the case notes of patients with lung cancer diagnosed by bronchoscopy.

(4) *Controlled versus uncontrolled trials.* A simple control group is one which omits the 'active treatment', but is otherwise identical in every way to the treatment group. Control groups can be more sophisticated and include patients treated with the 'standard' drug or combinations of new and old treatments. For a controlled trial to be valid, patients need to be allocated to the control and treatment groups in a randomized fashion.

Research involving patients must allow for the appreciable time required to complete protocols. For example, a prospective trial requires patients to be collected, the procedure studied to be completed, and then a suitable period allowed to elapse for review. Will this be a practical proposition for the amount of time you have available? If not, think again! You may have to restrict your plans to investigating a population that has already been documented and is awaiting continuing detailed analysis and study rather than starting entirely from scratch.

Experimental systems

Research using animal models is usually simpler and quicker but may appear less immediately clinically applicable. However, the scientist then has greater control over the experiment and subjects. In any case, new drugs or operative procedures must be tested on animal models before human trials. For such experiments, animal house facilities within, or available to, the department, are essential.

1. Animal houses are very expensive to set up. They must fulfil strict criteria for the humane management of animals controlled by law, and regulated (in the United Kingdom) by the Home Office.
2. Animals must be obtained from reputable suppliers, recognized as such by the Home Office.
3. Grants will normally allow you the recurrent costs of purchasing and maintaining the animal, but no more.
4. Overhead costs of animal house facilities, apart from board and lodging, usually cannot be met from a grant. In the United Kingdom, the dual support research system assumes that the laboratory receiving

the grant has the appropriate infrastructure to cover fundamentals such as animal care.

The study of cultured or otherwise isolated cells and tissues *in vitro* offers even greater powers of manipulation to the researcher. However, the results obtained are not necessarily applicable *in vivo* (in the living organism). In addition, the time necessary to prepare or grow the cells to conduct meaningful experiments varies with species of animal and with cell type. Tissue culture and other *in vitro* cellular work requires its own services and infrastructure within the department.

Ethical aspects

The ethics of working on human subjects is a large and important area of discussion. Most clinical trials must have prior approval from the local (usually hospital) ethical committee. It is important to determine at an early stage whether such approval is necessary and to initiate the procedures entailed. Most countries also have set criteria for carrying out drug trials. In the United Kingdom, a doctor or dentist is considered to be carrying out a clinical trial if he administers a medicinal product primarily to determine its effect. The doctor is then required to have a clinical trials certificate, or the manufacturer to hold a product licence.

A number of important regulations apply to animal experimentation to ensure that the most humane possible procedures are used in scientific work. The precise details by which these controls are applied vary with state or with country. They need to be studied carefully before contemplating animal research. In the United Kingdom, permission to perform animal experiments is covered by the Animal Procedures Act, under which licences are issued. Every individual researcher who wishes to conduct pro-cedures that fall outside a restricted range of manipulations must apply for a *Personal Licence*. A *Project Licence* is also issued to institutions which conduct scientific work. Applications for these require the project to be described, and the procedures on any living animal involved to be defined. Many institutions may already have project licences for your intended procedures for which further application is then not necessary. Information on Home Office Licences is obtainable from the Home Office Inspector responsible for the institution in which you propose to carry out your research.

In vitro studies of human tissues, including clinical material, require permission of the consultant in charge and written informed consent from the patients concerned.

Team vs individual work

Another consideration in choosing your research area is the amount of independence you want. There are a wide range of research laboratories. Large teams often have nearly everyone working on the same project. This has the advantage that your research is likely to be completed, but you may feel a very small cog in a big machine, and your name may only be one of many to appear on the research papers. Molecular biological research tends to be expensive and to involve large salaried teams. At the other extreme, working in some areas of cellular electrophysiology involves groups of as few as one or two scientists, and entails a lonelier existence. However, the research tends to be inexpensive, and the resulting published work involves few authors.

If you are conducting research as a postgraduate student or as a candidate for a higher medical degree, research expenses are usually covered by your supervisor's grant or by the laboratory. Accordingly, you will normally have to think relatively little about research costs other than your own applications for fellowships and studentships for your own personal support.

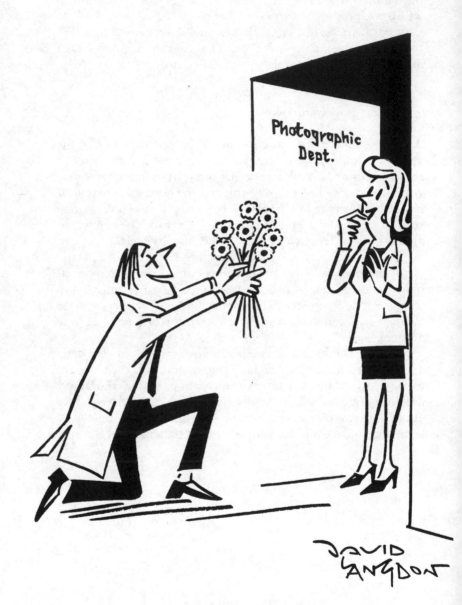

Grateful for assistance . . .

6

The first phase: getting started

Congratulations! You have now passed the major hurdles of making the decision to pursue research, and of following this decision through to the position where you are able to start. The remarks in this chapter primarily concern your fitting into, and learning to function in, this new environment.

A doctor in research

When you join a research laboratory, you will find yourself in a very different setting, with values distinct from those to which you are accustomed in the clinic or ward. You should try as quickly as possible to assimilate into the local scene. Even if the atmosphere in the laboratory is initially alien to you, this may reflect its tradition of research achievement just as the environment in a successful hospital promotes good clinical results. However, this does not mean a clinician does not have anything to offer a research environment. Some of the advantages you will have gained from a clinical background are as follows:

1. You will often be more realistic as to what to expect of others.
2. You will often have more social confidence and take more care in your dealings with others.
3. You will have a better sense of what can or cannot be achieved in limited time.
4. You will have gained more experience in making full use of available time.

41

5. You are more used to coping with more than one problem at a time.
6. You can often assist scientific colleagues with your ability to gain access to clinical material or knowledge.

However, there are a number of respects in which you must adapt.

1. You may be used to responding only to well-defined authority figures. In a research laboratory such individuals are not as clear-cut.
2. You may feel less confident at the bench. When starting out you will often find yourself embarrassingly out of touch with even elementary scientific procedures.
3. You may expect too much of the services of others.
4. You may be less accustomed to the longer-term planning that goes with research work.

Public relations

It follows that, as a fledgling researcher, you will depend greatly on the goodwill and the skills of others, and upon your relationships with key people. It is therefore important to establish and maintain a good rapport with everyone in the laboratory, whether scientific, technical, secretarial or administrative staff. You should aim to establish yourself as someone who is seen to be:

- diligent and productive;
- honest;
- courteous and reliable (for example, keep appointments and, if away, leave a note with a contact number or time of return on your desk);
- likely to benefit from any assistance given;
- grateful for assistance (for example, consider giving small Christmas presents, or at least cards, to your laboratory technician, photographic department and secretary);
- likely to acknowledge assistance received (for example, you might send copies of your publications with acknowledgements to those who gave you help).

An example of how good relations will smooth your time in research is your association with the photographic department. By placing small, simple, non-urgent requests with the department early, it is unlikely that you will need to harass the staff and you will be genuinely grateful when the material returns well in advance of your deadline. Furthermore, by establishing good rapport, the photographic staff would be more receptive when you have genuinely urgent or difficult demands, for example, in relation to your thesis deadline.

Self discipline

Research requires ample amounts of both self assurance and self control. You must be strict with yourself and be realistic with use of your time in relation to your ultimate aims. Research work is usually very individualistic: the success or failure of your project depends primarily upon yourself. Conversely, a lot of the other people in your laboratory are tied to more formal 'in laboratory' commitments, so you should also feel free to study in the library, write at home, or take a short sporting or holiday break if you know it will help you achieve your goal.

Maintaining clinical commitments

There is great value in maintaining a 'clinical string to your bow', particularly during longer stints in research (greater than six months). Consider the following suggestions, particularly if you desire ultimately to return to clinical medicine.

1. Choose the field of medicine you would like eventually to follow and, after discussing the matter with your supervisor, approach the relevant departmental head with an offer of your clinical services for a prescribed, fixed portion of the week. Some clinically attuned supervisors will do this for you. Be aware that it is unlikely you will be remunerated for this time.
2. Outpatient and operating sessions are valuable as they are well-circumscribed entities consistent with reliable planning of the rest of the week's research.
3. Try to make these clinical commitments relevant to your future interests or, best of all, to your current research. For example, if your laboratory project is a study of the effects of growth hormone on the healing of burns, a session a week assisting the plastic surgery team in theatre for a burns dressing and grafting list would be ideal. If your thesis is an electron microscopic investigation of lymphomas, you might consider attending the haematological or lymphoma outpatient clinic or ward round.
4. Obtain a contract, even if only an honorary one, from your employing body in the hospital setting out a specified number of clinical hours per week. In the United Kingdom at present all honorary clinical (even part-

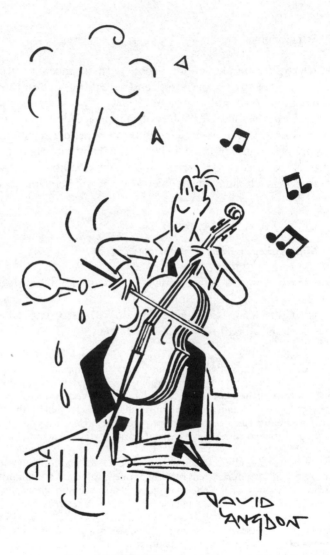

Extracurricular buffer . . .

time) jobs within the National Health Service are recognized as being full-time in terms of salary scales. For example, if you do three years as a part-time honorary Senior House Officer (SHO) during your research years, when you return to a full-time SHO position, you will be paid as a fourth-year SHO.

5. Similarly, your employer may pay Legal Medical Defence subscriptions.
6. Weekly Grand Rounds and clinical meetings are also invaluable for keeping in touch.

On the other hand, you should consider the following precautions.

1. Never get a 'bleeper'. One of the positive aspects of a period of research that you should enjoy is that you are a free agent. A bleeper by its very nature is a mental and emotional tie to a service, usually a hospital. It means people can contact you easily and at inconvenient times, for instance, during the middle of an intricate experiment.
2. Never be 'on call'. While on call you are responsible to patients and doctors. Although your periods of duty may be quiet, there will always be the potential for a distracting challenge at an inconvenient moment.
3. Be fastidiously firm with approaches from well-meaning people with requests for your services. Once you open the door to these demands, more and more approaches will flood in. Remember that your primary objective is to do your research and not to cover the hospital in case of clinical emergencies. If you maintain this firm line, your niche in the community will soon become established and respected.
4. Do not allow clinical obligations to take more than one day per week.

Extracurricular activities

Productivity of work towards a thesis increases with the time devoted to it. However, beyond a certain point, one tends to become less productive. Accordingly, include a variety of leisure activities while pursuing your research project to postpone this fall in productivity. In any case, some time taken well away from your research is necessary and beneficial. Extracurricular activities, whether they be sport, music, family, or a hobby, are good ways to achieve such a break and they positively influence morale, concentration and productivity. They also act as a 'buffer' for the times of minor mishap, disappointment and disaster that are inevitably associated with research.

Needless to say, there is a fine line between the beneficial and deleterious effects of extracurricular activities. Too much time and energy spent on other activities will detract from your research efforts.

Fitting in postgraduate medical examinations

Professional medical examinations, including the primary examinations of the Royal College of Physicians (MRCP) and Royal College of Surgeons (FRCS), those corresponding to other specialities, and the Foreign Medical Graduate Examination in the Medical Sciences (FMGEMS: an examination necessary for working as a doctor in the United States) are best completed early in one's postgraduate medical career. They require considerable study, and are best attempted during quiet jobs orientated toward the examination. In some cases, the early part of a period in research provides this opportunity. It is important to check the requirements and dates of these examinations with the relevant College or Board to determine if you can fit preparations for such examinations into your programme.

Getting started at the bench

Much of 'getting started' involves combining the ideas for research with the available facilities, time and literature to produce experimental results.

Early 'hands on' in the laboratory is essential. One approach to getting started at the bench: initially do not be too concerned about experimental design or what you are testing. Simply set yourself (or have your supervisor set you) a very simple problem in order to familiarize yourself with a particular laboratory technique or a group of related techniques that will be fundamental to your research. Once that technique is mastered, move to the next in the sequence, all the while contemplating how you could use these techniques to test an interesting hypothesis, and/or how you can improve the technique. Once you know roughly what works, how easy or difficult it is, and how long it takes, you can set yourself simple hypotheses to test, and plan some experiments. While doing this, continue to review the literature at times when you are unable to be by the bench.

However, research students tend to devote too much attention to the literature. It is much easier to go into the library and read some journals than it is to walk into an unfamiliar laboratory and begin an experiment. You could spend forever reviewing the literature; it is important, but stifling. Obsessive reading fosters a negative frame of mind and makes you think about what you cannot do, not what you can do.

Choosing laboratory techniques

Much time in the early stages of pursuing research is spent assessing the facilities and techniques that are available to you.
A *useful technique* is one that:

- is regularly performed in your laboratory
- is reproducible
- has controls already in existence
- is easy to set up
- produces rapid results that you can assess
- produces simple and unambiguous results.

A *less useful technique* is likely to have one or more of these disadvantages:

- untried
- not reproducible
- difficult to perform and expensive in money and time
- takes long to produce results (months/years)
- produces ambiguous results.

A supervisor experienced in the techniques that you employ and the ways of approaching your problem is particularly helpful. You will still have a feeling of independence if your project is close enough to your supervisor's own work to interest him, but distant enough so that you are pursuing an interest of your own.

Planning experiments

When planning your experiments consider the following suggestions.

1. *Don't be too ambitious:* the first experiment, carefully done and with small numbers, often works. It is when you complicate the experimental

design with extra groups, variables and numbers that it falls apart and the data become impossible to interpret!

2. *Analyse results as you go along:* proper and prompt analysis, although initially apparently time-consuming, is ultimately more efficient as it allows the researcher to plan more effective subsequent experiments.

3. *Avoid heroics:* start with simple experiments that work and gradually progress upwards. Allow time for unforeseen but inevitable disasters (for example, broken equipment, unavailable chemicals).

4. *Number of projects:* have more than one activity running at any given time. Most experiments entail periods of waiting, and it is useful to 'dove-tail' several of these together in order to use your time most effectively, but not to the point where you end up with distractions, confusion and mistakes.

5. *Weekly routine:* consider establishing a weekly routine. For instance, you might carry out a planned experiment early in the week or early in the day. Analyse the previous week's results midweek, and prepare for next week's activities late week. Have set days and times for your clinical and extracurricular activities.

6. *Label your samples, containers and computer disks:* identify all materials with your name, the date of purchase and/or purpose, preferably in a colour specific to you. Keep them together in the refrigerator, freezer or shelf, so that they can be found and identified unambiguously when in a hurry.

Keeping careful notes

Above all, keep careful notes of procedures and results in your laboratory notebook. A hard-backed, lined exercise book is an invaluable aid to planning, carrying out and analysing your experiments.

1. *Date* each day's work.
2. Write the *aim* of the experiment.
3. *Materials:* record the model, manufacturer and code number of equipment and sources of chemicals used as you go. This procedure saves much time and energy later on.
4. *Methods:* include full notes and related citations for all your procedures.
5. Make a note when you alter a standard procedure, with the date and the exact details of the alteration. Similarly, do likewise should you subsequently return to the original method.
6. Always write or stick the *results* directly into the book.
7. *Analysis:* when something goes wrong (e.g. mixing-up tubes, adding the wrong chemical) write it in. Something that appears obvious at the time will be forgotten months or years later.
8. Number the pages and set up an *index* at the back of your book (or in your personal computer) so that results and procedures can be found easily.

Consulting a statistician

It is beyond the scope of this book to discuss statistical analysis of data in any great detail. Nearly all medical researchers have some acquaintance with basic statistics, but there is no easy way to acquire insight into all the important statistical concepts and principles. Furthermore, statistics is not as 'cut and dried' a subject as you might expect. Good statistical analysis requires common sense and judgement, as well as a repertoire of formal techniques. It is often not possible to prescribe one statistical method for all the data analysis bearing upon a given problem.

It is therefore advisable to consult a statistician at an *early* stage while planning your experiments, particularly if your project requires analysis of lots of figures. Doing this will result in additional advantages.

1. You begin a professional relationship with the expert which will continue and develop as the project unfolds.
2. The statistician can advise you on the sample sizes you are likely to require to make the experiment or study statistically valid. Mistakes in experimental design often cannot be rectified retrospectively when analysing data.
3. The statistician may suggest a method of data collection that will make statistical analysis simpler.
4. The statistician will direct you to an appropriate choice of statistical method, and may arrange access to the appropriate statistical software for later analysis.
5. You will have greater confidence in your statistical methods if your examiners or referees criticize them.

Setting out

By now one would hope that you are now up and running, and that you have found some methods that work and some hypotheses to test. These are heady days, for you feel you are getting a grip on the 'tools of science' and it is now a matter of putting them into practice. Before getting too carried away, you might consider some cautionary words of advice, that may save time and problems later.

1. *Record all experimental details.* Photograph all your interesting histological sections, cell cultures, operative techniques and so on. Consider an instamatic or polaroid camera for 'instant' pictures of your results.

2. *Set yourself flow charts* to map out how you have progressed and where you are heading.
3. *Continually assess.* Make sure you understand the results you are get-ting. If not why not? Write your thoughts down. Don't necessarily dis-miss odd or 'quirky' results. They may end up by being the most interest-ing.
4. *Think ahead.* Plan for unforeseen circumstances, and for foreseen delays. For example, apply for your animal licence well in advance while work-ing out the details of your experiment. Order required equipment and chemicals well before you actually need them. By the time these arrive, you may be ready to proceed.
5. *Be flexible.* Although planning is laudable, you should never be so rigid that you cannot follow a new avenue or drop an unrewarding one.

Research reports

Many faculty boards, funding bodies and supervisors ask for peri-odic progress reports from research students on their work. While this may seem annoying and constricting while you are in full experi-mental flight, they do have several important functions. These include:

* focussing your mind on which hypotheses you are testing and how you are testing them;
* giving you practice at scientific writing;
* providing a useful store of organized information to be used when you come to write up your thesis.

Following the literature

An important, indeed vital, part of your thesis is the review of pre-vious publications in your field of study and in its related topics. Such a literature review has a number of essential functions.

1. It provides you with an idea of the current state of knowledge in the field and enables you to identify possible gaps where further work might be of value.
2. It details the research techniques employed in the study.
3. It will form an important part of two portions of the thesis, the Introduc-tion and the Discussion (see Chapter 11).

Do not try to carry out an exhaustive literature search before you start your own experimental investigations. First of all, this will depress you to see just how much is already known about your topic and, secondly, following up the resulting bibliography will take up such a horrendous amount of time that your available period of research will be spent mainly in the library! Rather, a preliminary review is often better based on selected papers and/or monographs which your supervisor will provide. They should be enough to get you started with the aims of the project and details of the techniques that you will be using. Most, if not all, of these should be well known to your supervisor and other members of the laboratory staff.

Reviewing the literature will continue all through your research period. Appropriately directed reading will draw your attention to fresh opportunities for experimental study of which you might not otherwise have been aware. Conversely, areas which you might otherwise have pursued relentlessly may turn out to be of marginal interest or already intensively studied, not justifying a time-consuming investigation. You should continue to follow developments in the literature after submitting your thesis while awaiting your oral examination, even if this involves a wait of several months. It would be unfortunate if you missed an important review article or publication in a well-read journal which appeared just a few weeks before your viva and which your examiners had read or, worse still, which one of them had actually written!

At present there are more than 10 000 medical journals published annually, and each year the number increases. Fortunately, indexing and abstracting services have existed for more than a century and these make literature searches in medical fields easier than in many other disciplines. In particular, computer searches of recent publications in a particular medical area can be done relatively easily.

Medical libraries differ greatly between themselves in organization. Perhaps the single most important thing to do is to know your own library and particularly its staff. Even small libraries usually have indexing journals, and either a computer terminal or some other access to computer searching facilities.

Important sources of references include the following.

(1) *Index Medicus*. This has indexed medical periodicals since 1879. It appears monthly with a cumulator at the end of the year making up fourteen volumes annually. It indexes more than 2500 international medical and paramedical journals by both author and subject. If you have not used this before, it is worth persuading your medical librarian to discuss with you the use of this invaluable tool.

(2) *Excerpta Medica*. This is currently classified into over 40 sections (e.g. cancer section 16, plastic surgery section 34). It covers some 3500 journals, and the particular volume relevant to your work can be most useful.

(3) *Computer searches*. Many libraries now have facilities, for example through Medlars and Medline, to search the literature appearing over a given time span by author, title, keyword, or combinations of these. Some libraries even make available self-access Index Medicus stored on disks, which can be searched or printed out by the student. Alternatively, at a cost, you could use a modem to gain access to a national scientific literature store. If your library has access to computer searches, and once you have found an appropriate combination of keywords, it is often very helpful to arrange to obtain a monthly update to your initial computer search.

Two useful books to help you are:

- Welch, J. & King, T. A. (1985). *Searching the Medical Literature. A guide to Printed and Online Sources*. London: Chapman & Hall Medical.
- Jenkins, S. (1987). *Medical Libraries: A User Guide*. London: British Medical Association.

Compiling references

You should photocopy your important references for personal use. Number and record their titles in a form corresponding to that required in your final thesis. For example, write out the title of the paper as well as the journal reference, and include all authors in full; do not abbreviate authors names to '*et al.*' at this stage (see Chapter 11). You can store your references either on a database system if you have a personal computer or by using a box file with lined cards. Put on the top of each card a note such as 'historical' or 'methodology' for easy sorting and file the cards alphabetically by first author.

Personal computers

Personal computers are becoming cheaper, more powerful and their programs progressively easier to use. They offer useful research facilities, including word processing, graphics, reference storage and handling, and storage and statistical analysis of data. Until recently, preparing a thesis would entail writing out the text long-hand, taking it to a typist chapter by chapter, submitting the typed copy to the supervisor, and then correcting, rewriting, and collating it before taking it back to the typist and going through this process again several times. Writing your thesis on a personal computer simplifies many of these steps and has a number of advantages.

1. Complete control over writing and presentation of your thesis.
2. The ability to modify, rearrange, and add to the text at any time: this makes it easy to draft your thesis in parallel with doing your research.
3. The ability to print multiple copies any time.
4. Scientific papers and whole theses can be sent to a colleague on a relatively lightweight disk.
5. The thesis text can easily be modified when writing scientific papers and vice versa.
6. Once use of the computer system is mastered, subsequent papers become easier to produce.
7. Keeping track of all references.
8. You can offset the cost of having your thesis typed against the cost of the computer system.

The disadvantages of using a personal computer include:

1. You need to learn to type (although you could purchase a 'learn to type' program).
2. The process of mastering the machine and the program is initially time-consuming.
3. It is probably slower than having a professional type your thesis on his/her computer. (You could, of course, arrange to have this done, and use your own computer to manipulate the text at a later date.)
4. If your data are not regularly 'backed up' on a spare storage disk or other medium, malfunctions in the software operating system or the machine could result in large sections of your work being lost.

Background computer information

If you decide to use a personal computer, it would be wise to begin to do so early in your research period. There is much to learn and it is impracticable to leave this to a few weeks before your final thesis submission. Most laboratories and departments have computing facilities. This is a good place to start, particularly as it does not involve any expense on your part. Eventually, you may wish for the greater flexibility and freedom of your own personal computer. Microcomputing systems have become popular particularly since the introduction of the personal computer by IBM in 1981. Since then, some 15 million models of essentially the same design have been sold in the US alone. The less sophisticated versions of these and similar machines, while not particularly fast or glamorous in relation to computing power now available, are competent general-purpose computers adequate for most writing, filing and small database requirements. Apart from the processor component of the computing system itself, you need to consider a number of things.

(1) *Memory:* most software programs require at least 128 kilobytes (128K) of random access memory within the computer. Computer systems with at least 640K are preferable.

(2) *Disk drives:* it is possible to operate a computer system with just one disk drive but this entails frequent and tedious switching of disks in and out of the machine, particularly when copying files and programs. It is considerably more convenient to have two drives, one for the program being run, and one for the data being collected. Even more useful is a hard disk, a storage device made of ceramic or aluminium, which is mounted inside a sealed drive unit and holds many times more information than will fit into a floppy disk. A hard disk will store all the programs that you would normally need for your research. It will eliminate much of the tedious switching of disks, and offer a substantial improvement in processing speed.

(3) *Monitors:* monochrome monitors to display text and graphics are relatively cheap and of good resolution.

(4) *Printers:* a 24-pin dot matrix printer is an inexpensive means of producing draft documents. If you obtain one that can also print in a 'letter quality' or 'near letter quality' mode, this may also be adequate for printing your thesis.

Besides word-processing, microcomputers offer other applications.

(1) *Database software:* microcomputers, preferably those with hard disks, can store and manipulate large amounts of information, including clinical records.

(2) *Statistical programs:* small, simple statistical packages such as OXSTAT can be run on microcomputers with less than even 720 kilobytes of memory. Larger, more sophisticated programs, such as SPSS (Statistical Package for the Social Sciences), originally designed for mainframe computers, are now available for those more recent microcomputer models with at least 20 megabytes of memory.

(3) *Graphics programs:* scientific graphics packages used to drive

a plotter or high-quality printer, such as a laser printer, can be very useful for the rapid preparation of tables and graphs.

(4) *Reference handling:* programs designed for storing, handling and formatting references for various journals are available. Alternatively, one could use standard word-processing or database programs.

Dictaphones

If you are accustomed to composing letters using a small, hand-held tape recorder (dictaphone), or if you find that you can compose much faster by thinking aloud, it may be worth purchasing a dictaphone and a typist's tape recorder with foot pedals and headphones. You can then dictate to yourself in almost any situation and then type the material into your computer at a more convenient time, using the tape recorder.

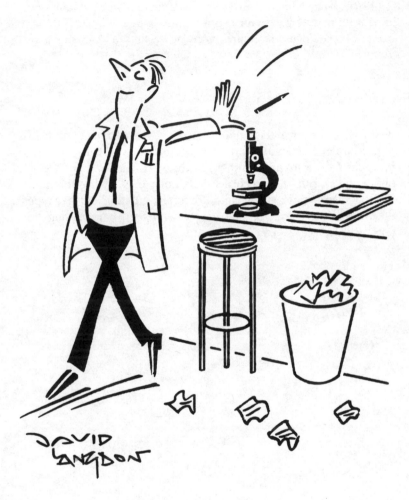

React creatively . . .

7

The second phase: frustration

React creatively to failure

Inevitably the heady days of early successes, new techniques and new equipment come to a resounding end when the inherent weaknesses of the procedure, equipment, hypothesis, approach, or even the problem you have set yourself become manifest. Setbacks and failures are inevitable. Being aware of this, and realistic about it, will help you to cope. It is important not to take such events too seriously, but to treat them in an analytical, almost detached fashion, as yet another problem to solve.

In addition, it is important to be clear that if you do not obtain positive results, or the findings that you expected, this need not be identified with failure. Disproving a particular point conclusively can be as constructive and scientific an outcome as proving a hypothesis. However, it is genuinely disheartening when experiments do not seem to work at all. Individuals vary a great deal in the way they react to such obstacles. Here are some alternatives.

Repeat the same procedure

1. Do this when you think the procedure you have adopted is fundamentally sound.
2. This course of action is desirable provided that you re-examine the situation and assess the problem before you repeat.

3. This course of action is inappropriate if it involves repeated uncritical attempts without your thinking about the reasons for the lack of success.

Alter the procedure or method of attack

1. Try this if your original response was tentative, and you can reinterpret the problem and attempt a new approach.
2. This course of action is appropriate if the altered tactics are based on a careful analysis of the problem and the previous method of attack is also given due assessment and criticism.
3. This approach is undesirable if the new method is adopted thoughtlessly.

Modify your goal

1. Try this if an alternative goal is available, or if you no longer expect the original goal to be attainable. Alternatively, you may feel the original goal was not a high priority in your overall project.
2. This decision is desirable if:
     i. the new goal satisfies the same needs as the original one;
    ii. the new goal leads to learning something useful;
   iii. the original goal is unimportant or not feasible.
3. This action is inadvisable if:
     i. the substitute goal is also unrealistic;
    ii. you are retreating when reasonable further effort will result in success;
   iii. the substitute goal actually unbalances the overall plan of your project.

Give up the procedure or goal

1. You are likely to select this course of action if you do not expect to succeed in your original goal, or if you think the goal is unimportant, or the means to achieve it are too difficult.
2. An alternative is to return to the problem later in the project.
3. This course of action is undesirable if reasonable further effort will, in fact, ensure success.

Quire clearly, the appropriate course of action varies with circumstances, and good judgement is necessary. In situations like this, your supervisor will be particularly helpful. He will have more experience and a better intuitive 'feel' of what is or is not going to work. You can also help yourself by keeping a well-annotated and full practical book. Finally, altering one's goals should not necessarily be seen as merely an 'easy way out'. Goals should remain flexible, since often new and more interesting goals will present themselves as work progresses.

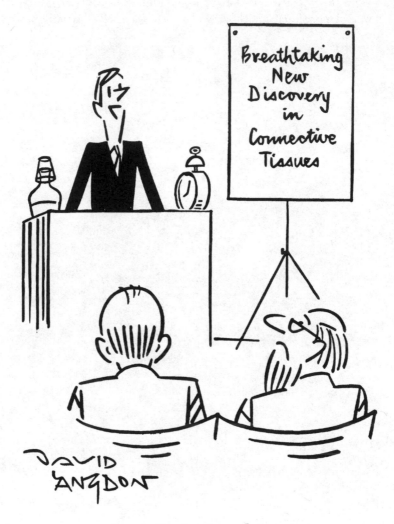

Presentation . . .

8

The third phase: as results arrive

Introduction

The 'results' phase is the most rewarding. However, it often arrives gradually and insidiously as your methods and thoughts develop and crystallize. It may only be on reflection that you appreciate how much has been achieved. The priority now is to keep up the momentum. You will by now have established patterns and methods of using your time. Stick to them and 'crunch out' the results! Once again, we emphasize the importance of analysing your results early and as you go along. It is not appropriate to place undigested records of your findings in a pile to be sifted through during the writing phase months or even years hence.

If you continually fail to obtain meaningful results or the methods are still not working, you must seriously consider changing direction, and this may involve the research project, laboratory or supervisor.

Once a reasonable set of results are to hand, you may wish to present them to your colleagues and peers for comments and criticism. Indeed, many programmes require postgraduate students to present their findings at departmental seminars. You may be encouraged by your supervisor to go further and display your work to a wider view, possibly through presentation at a meeting, verbally, by poster, or both, or by submission of a paper for publication.

Presentations at meetings

There is a hierarchy of fora at which you can display your work, ranging from informal discussion in the laboratory to giving a paper at an international meeting. These can be graded in ascending order as follows.

1. Seminar in your department.
2. Local meeting of a specialist society in your field, e.g. the London Connective Tissue Society Meeting.
3. National meeting of professional or academic societies, e.g. British Connective Tissue Society.
4. International Conferences, covering a particular interest, e.g. International Symposium on Basement Membranes.
5. Major International Conferences, e.g. Gordon Conferences.

The advantages of presenting at a meeting include:

1. making contact with, and gaining recognition from, other researchers in your field;
2. securing priority for your work;
3. getting practice in presenting work, and answering criticisms and questions (particularly useful for your approaching oral examination on your thesis);
4. keeping up to date with progress in your field through contact with other participants and attending their presentations.

Verbal presentations

When preparing to present a paper before a scientific audience, consider the following.

1. Check that your topic being presented is within the scope of the meeting.
2. If possible, check what the other presenters will be covering and to what depth, to avoid repetition and/or lack of background information.
3. Presentations should be rehearsed against the clock in front of one, or preferably more, colleagues. There is usually a time limit on presentations. It is very frustrating to be stopped by the meeting's chairperson 30 seconds before one reaches the climax of one's talk.
4. Check what audio visual aids (e.g. single or dual carousel projectors) are available, and whether they are compatible with the form of your presented material.
5. Check how the pointer and slide controller work before the start of the day's meeting,

Poster presentations

An increasing proportion of conferences now invite poster, and not only verbal, presentations. Often specific times are allocated at the meeting for presentation and discussion of posters. They are a useful way for a beginner to learn how to display information. Here is a list of hints on ensuring an effective poster.

1. Ensure that the poster conforms with the specifications laid down by the organizing committee.
2. Try to present only one short central message. If you have a lot of material to present, or more than one message, submit two posters.
3. Make sure that you get advice from your medical illustration department about how the lettering and illustrations are prepared and displayed.
4. Keep text to a minimum.
5. Make sure that you state a clear-cut conclusion.

Funding your visit

If the meeting is to be held in another city or overseas, you will naturally incur travel and accommodation expenses. If your paper or poster has been accepted, this is not usually a problem. There will then probably be a departmental, university, hospital or district authority fund which will cover the costs of your travel and (modest!) hotel or hostel bills. In some cases, if your work involves collaboration with a pharmaceutical or scientific instrument company, they may provide such funding.

Publishing papers

It is during this time that you may have acquired sufficient data to begin to publish. Your supervisor will be the best person to advise when and where. There are several advantages of publishing at this stage.

1. The exercise will concentrate your thoughts, reveal areas of inadequacy in your work, and areas for further testing.
2. You will gain practice at scientific writing.
3. Most journals, whether they accept or reject your paper, will return copies of referees' comments. These usually contain important criticisms

which range from grammatical and lettering mistakes, to omissions in your review of the literature and suggestions for further investigations. It is a great benefit to consider these criticisms in your own time, rather than in the heat of a thesis viva!
4. Many of the figures, tables and graphs you will prepare for submission for publication will be useful again in your thesis.

Choice of journal

It can be difficult to decide on the particular journal to which you might submit your paper. Advice from your supervisor will be most helpful. Considerations include:

1. the quality of your paper, and the significance of its scientific contribution;
2. your potential audience: whether you are aiming for a large medical and/or scientific audience, or a group of specialists.

Journals vary in a number of important respects.

1. Circulation: size of the readership.
2. Width of readership: international, national, regional or local.
3. Content and interest: scientifically orientated or clinically orientated.
4. Breadth of interest: the degree of specialization of the journal.

The last point is exemplified below for medical journals.

Category	Example of journal
Broad scientific	*Nature*
Medicine in general	*New England Journal of Medicine*
Speciality medical	*Journal of Bone and Joint Surgery*
Subspeciality medical	*Journal of Hand Surgery*

A similar pattern exists for more scientifically orientated journals.

Category	Example of journal
Broad scientific	*Nature*
A field of science	*Biochemical Journal*
Speciality in that field	*Lipid Research*
Subspeciality	*Prostaglandins*

Submitting a paper

A paper is usually submitted typed double-spaced on white A4 paper with 1 inch margins, in the following sequence.

1. Front page with title of paper, and names of authors and laboratories, addresses of authors, address for correspondence and for reprint requests, and three to five keywords.
2. Abstract or summary on a separate page.
3. The main bulk of the paper which comprises: Introduction, Materials and Methods, Results, and Discussion (see Chapter 11).
4. Acknowledgements.
5. References, beginning on a separate page and still double-spaced.
6. Legends to figures: a new page for each legend.

Before you send off your paper, make sure you have followed the 'Instructions to authors' from the relevant journal. These regulations are often printed in the first issue of that year, or even in every issue. Find a paper from a recent issue of the journal to use as a model. Your submission should include the following.

1. The required number of copies of the paper.
2. The required number of figures. Usually 15 cm × 10 cm prints, labelled in pencil on the back with the first author's name, figure number and the top of the figure indicated.
3. Any publications quoted as 'in press', or that may be difficult for the referees to locate easily.
4. A short covering letter.

Most journals will acknowledge your submission within two weeks. If the paper is obviously inappropriate for the journal, the manuscript will be returned a few weeks later.

Steps leading to publication

If the journal decides to have the paper refereed, you may wait two to nine months for a reply. On receiving referee's reports, the editor will do one of the following.

1. Reject your paper outright.
2. Accept the paper for publication, provided that you attend to the suggestions of the referees. These may range from minor omissions, to an extra experiment or two. When revising the paper in response to these requests, it is worth while to list each of the alterations you have made, corresponding to each of the reviewer's comments in your reply.
3. Accept the paper for publication, without further alterations.

Once the final version of your paper has been accepted, the publisher may make minor adjustments and will set the text according to the printed style of the journal. Most publishers will send page proofs to you for final checking. You should particularly check the details of you and your fellow authors! You will also be provided with a request form for reprints. Journals vary in their generosity with supplying reprints. Order at least 100. Your department will usually pay any costs. Some journals additionally levy page charges to cover printing costs, particularly for colour photographs.

The time from submission to publication is often long (up to eighteen months or even two years). In general, weekly journals that have large international subscriptions (e.g. *Nature*, *The Lancet*) publish most promptly (sometimes in less than six months). Specialized journals that may only put out several issues a year are the slowest.

The author nominated to deal with reprint requests may be inundated with requests from all over the world, often from countries with poor library and photocopying facilities.

Securing your future

If you have not done so already, you should think about your next career position at this stage. You may now have a good indication of what you will gain from your research and so can convey this in your applications to future employers. It is a great advantage to know where and when you will be going next. Furthermore, if you manage to secure a position that will follow your research project before the writing-up stage, you will be free from employment uncertainties, and be able to devote your time more effectively to completing your project.

Towards the end of the 'Results' phase, during the process of submitting papers or as you begin to write up your results, you will become aware of the necessity to perform, often tedious, control experiments. The purpose of these experiments is to convince yourself and your readers (including examiners) that your methods were valid, and your results reproducible and not a 'one-off' phenomenon. These experiments should be completed as soon as possible.

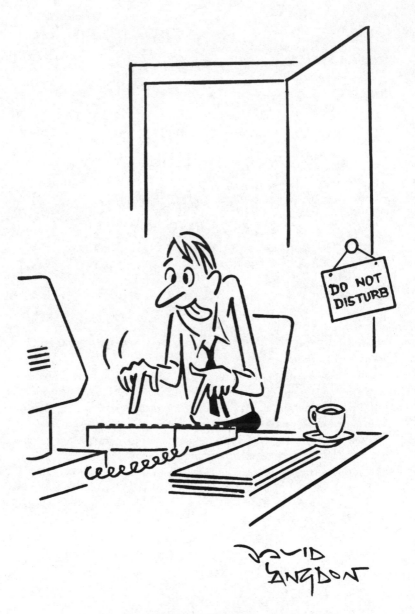

Writing the thesis . . .

9

The fourth phase: writing the thesis

Time and place

There are two extreme approaches to timing when it comes to writing up a thesis. Most students will reach a compromise between the two. You could start writing your dissertation only after completing all your experimental work. However, it is preferable to write a sequence of short accounts in the course of your project as you gather results and draw conclusions. Writing periodic progress reports and papers as circumscribed parts of your project become completed can form part of this process.

Writing continuously as you collect data has a number of advantages. It reduces the amount of pressure on you as you approach your thesis deadline, and encourages the good habit of reviewing and analysing data soon after they are obtained. In any case, writing as you go helps fill in periods where you are unable to do experiments; for example, when equipment is being serviced or repaired. Observing your dissertation as it gradually evolves, rather than anticipating the massive task of writing it, builds morale. Additionally, working some of your findings into publications will improve your chances of obtaining your next job, as then you will have something to show for your work. Finally, the time at which you decide to stop laboratory work and devote your time entirely to writing becomes less critical.

However, circumstances or inclination may lead you to leave any substantial writing to the end. Alternatively, you may persuade yourself that this course takes a smaller absolute amount of time, or that you feel you can better keep your data in mind, as a whole, if you allocated large stretches of time entirely to writing.

The timing of your writing up will in turn determine where you do it. If you draft your thesis in the course of your experimental work, it is likely that you will have time to write up your thesis while still in the laboratory. If you leave writing until you have completed all conceivable experiments, it is likely you will only get around to writing after you have left your laboratory. Most research students will take the most sensible choice of doing something in between.

If you get to do your writing up while still in your laboratory, you will be conveniently close to the equipment and chemicals you used and to advice from colleagues. Additionally, your supervisor may be close at hand to comment on your work as you progress. However, your colleagues still doing laboratory work may find your presence an obstruction; laboratories are often pushed for space, and other workers may also need the computer or word processor which you are using. Finally, you may be more likely to be interrupted while in a busy laboratory.

Conversely there are some advantages to completing your writing away from the laboratory. You will be free from all distractions of a normal laboratory, and you may be able to look at your work more objectively. However, you then may not have some important sources of information to hand: you may realize while writing that you have forgotten your brand of fetal calf serum or the settings on your centrifuge. Additionally, depending on temperament, there are more distractions from composing when away from the laboratory.

A final possibility, which you should certainly try to avoid, is that you only get the opportunity to write up your thesis after you have left the laboratory, and you have already started your next employment. You will then combine the disadvantages of both the above options. You will not have the benefit of being near scientific advice and assistance, yet be readily distracted by colleagues in your new place of work, who may not be in the least interested in your previous work. You may also irritate your new senior colleagues or employer in being distracted by a commitment you still have to fulfil.

Furthermore, if you then take up an appointment which has a heavy clinical load, the quite considerable time you need to write up your thesis may just not be there. Finally, in what time there is available, you will find that you are tired, distracted, and all too often interrupted by the telephone or by your 'bleep'.

Winding up experimental work

It is very important, even while writing up, to allocate some time to return to the bench for some (usually minor) tidying up experiments, for example, those extra controls that the referee wants before your paper is published. One approach would be to keep one day or half day a week working in the laboratory as you are writing, at least at the outset. You will then remain familiar with the layout of the laboratory and its facilities, and be in touch with any changes. A return to the laboratory after a prolonged absence can be very frustrating when all the chemicals have moved, and you have forgotten the minor intricacies of a particular method. The pressures of completing a thesis will amplify these frustrations.

When do you stop experimental work completely?

This is difficult to decide. There is a natural tendency for your supervisor to keep you hard at experiments; after all, to him your work is often part of a continuing project. On the other hand, students usually underestimate by at least 50% the time needed to perform particular tasks. This is especially the case for writing up theses. You will be surprised how long important processes, such as reading, printing out drafts, preparing illustrations, and editing will take. Delays, of course, can be reduced by careful planning and setting up early on.

One rule of thumb is that if you have written and have had accepted two substantial papers (not just abstracts), or have sufficient data for two such papers that you expect will be accepted by reputable refereed journals, you have enough material for your MD or PhD thesis, and can turn from experimental work to writing up.

Planning your thesis

Completing a thesis is a formidable task. You should start planning and thinking about your thesis from the first day of your research project. It will fill your life for the duration of your research. In this connection, always have a notebook handy. You will be amazed at the times when insights about your research problem, or a minor flash of inspiration relevant to the dissertation, will occur. If you write down such thoughts, you can return to them later in a more objective frame of mind.

If you continually bear in mind the approach and organization you are trying to develop for your thesis, it will help you greatly in emerging with a clear picture of how you wish to organize your thesis, at a relatively early stage. This is a situation where a personal computer is particularly useful. Keeping your outline on a file on your personal computer will encourage you to develop and improve your thesis outline. To see the form of your thesis developing with time is encouraging and promotes work towards a more cohesive thesis. A personal computer is also often convenient for storing technical and scientific information for manipulation, amendment, expansion and retrieval at a later date.

Format of your thesis

As material, results and ideas develop, you will get a progressively better idea of the form your thesis will take. In addition, the nature of your thesis should be influenced by the following.

(1) *Studying the university regulations*

Obtain the regulations for your degree in your university, and read and digest them, particularly the regulations governing preparation of theses and abstracts submitted for your particular degree.

(2) *Considering ways of organizing the material*

In theory, you are relatively free to write your thesis as you like, provided that you follow university regulations. In practice, it is probably best to conform to tested ways of presenting work. There are two main possibilities, depending on the nature of your project. You could write your dissertation in a single coherent unit, organized into Introduction, Methods, Results, and Discussion (see Chapter 11). Alternatively you could write up separate components of your work in sequence, each in turn divided into separate Introduction, Methods, Results, and Discussion, with a final common Discussion chapter which ties them all together.

(3) *Inspecting past successful theses completed by others*

It is helpful to examine as early as possible theses written in similar areas by your predecessors. These are often available in your university or departmental library. If you do this at an early stage, you will then be most influenced by appearance and least by content! You may also be able to locate, and pay particular attention to, your supervisor's own thesis. This exercise will illustrate to you ways to organize and lay out your material, and mistakes you may wish to avoid. Make notes on, or photocopy for your records, the appealing features of each thesis. You could use a particular thesis as an overall model, and aim to improve it by incorporating attractive features noted elsewhere.

(4) *Considering the length of different sections*

It is helpful to have a clear idea in your mind of the relative allocation of pages to:
Introduction
Methods
Results
Discussion
This is the usual form in which scientific material is organized (see Chapter 11). The relative emphasis of each aspect will vary with project, and the amount and nature of your results. One approach might be to first decide upon your expected overall thesis length (giving due note to the regulations, and examining other theses), then allocating 30–40% of the pages to the Results with as much as needed for the Methods. Divide the remaining pages roughly equally between the Introduction and Discussion. Then modify this basic scheme as needs become clearer, as you do your writing up.

Order of writing

The following is a frequently adopted order of writing.

1. Materials
2. Methods
3. Results
4. Introduction

5. Discussion
6. Abstract
7. Title, keywords
8. References

Advice on each of these sections is given in Chapter 11. This sequence starts you off writing about simple hard facts, then subsequently progresses through observations, analysis, and conjectures, to abstractions.

Photocopying facilities

Access to a photocopier is essential for research students. Find one or several as soon as possible. Ideally, you would want to have access to the following.

1. A photocopier that is cheap to use and easily accessible from your library, for photocopying references and day-to-day work. British and international copyright law permits you to make one copy of a certain proportion of a published work for personal use.
2. A photocopier that is cheap and easily accessible to your laboratory, for photocopying results. It is a very good policy to give a copy of all your results to your supervisor for the simple reason that, if your own copies get lost, he will save the day!
3. A high-quality photocopier, to produce your final thesis.

Preparing illustrations

When planning your thesis, it often helps first to decide upon the illustrations, including graphs and tables, that you wish to include and the order in which you wish to present them. This will help organize your writing. You should check the university regulations governing the format of illustrations and their preparation at the outset of your project. With this in mind, you should make a conscious decision at an early stage as to how you will label your graphs, what units you will use and how you want to express them. Make a note of this style and stick to it. All your illustrations will then be acceptable to university regulations from the outset, and this will help avoid re-drawing and re-lettering later. Also make sure that in the labels on the illustrations you use the same abbreviations, mathematical symbols, and general style as in the text and captions.

(1) *Doing it yourself* by hand is the most time-consuming, but you

can then control precisely how you present your data, and when you complete the work. You will need a fair amount of practice, persistence, and patience. You will require certain basic materials, including $100g/m^2$ transparent drawing paper; drawing board and pens; tracing paper and lettering stencils, or access to lettering machines.

(2) *By computer:* if you have a department microcomputer with plotter, with the necessary software and hardware, this would offer an extremely convenient way of preparing tables and graphs.

(3) Very well-endowed departments may allow you access to the professional *departmental illustrator*. If you are in this fortunate position, you should introduce yourself to the departmental illustrator early in your project. Establish rapport by first submitting simple small projects with long deadlines. Get any material to the illustrator considerably earlier than you require it, even if it means having some results drawn up that may be relevant to your thesis months or even years in advance. The worst scenario is to hand in all your illustrations the week before the thesis is due to go to be bound, without giving the illustrator advance warning.

Do not prepare illustrations in such a hurry that you make careless mistakes. These mistakes often stay unnoticed until a much later stage (for example, as you are about to post the proofs to a journal).

Photographic work

Unless you are particularly good at home processing, it is advisable to arrange all the printing of your illustrations through your photographic department. Six 15 cm × 10 cm (or 20 cm × 15 cm) prints of each illustration is a good number to start with, along with one 35 mm slide. This usually gives you enough prints both to submit for publication to a journal, and for your thesis. The slide would be useful for a future presentation at a lecture or seminar. If you need extra, usually smaller, versions of photomicrographs for your thesis, it is probably best to leave these until your thesis is nearer completion. You may then wish to magnify, or reduce or collage them into part of a larger illustration, and so on.

It is more convenient and tidier to photocopy prints of line drawings and graphs for your thesis, rather than pasting in original prints. High-quality photocopying machines are very useful for enlarging and reducing drawings.

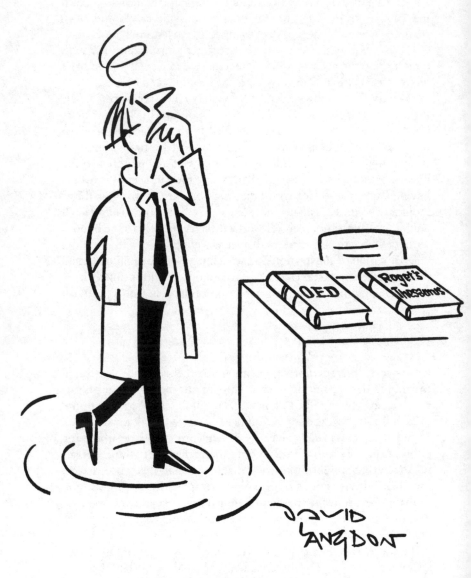

Decide what to say . . .

10

Scientific writing

How you express yourself in writing profoundly influences your reader's and, more importantly, your examiner's impression of your work. A small number of talented, experienced and much practised writers are able to write quickly and fluently, but most of us require considerable effort to make our writings acceptable. The brief remarks in this section may provide some help on how to compose scientific prose and indicate some of the reasons why a given piece of scientific writing may be unsatisfactory. However, they cannot replace more substantial volumes on the use of English, to which the reader must refer if he or she wants more definitive details.

Decide what to say

The first step in writing is to be absolutely clear as to what you want to say. The best English in the world will not compensate for a writer with nothing to report. Note down in a rough, not necessarily logical, fashion a list of the points you wish to make. They can then be ordered later, or in the course of writing.

Decide how it needs to be said

Determine how your writing needs to be organized. University regulations and past theses need to be consulted.

Organize your thoughts

Any reasoned argument requires a logical sequence. Consequently, before writing any paper or chapter, you should order your thoughts to create a logical outline of your subject matter.

1. Break down each chapter or section of your planned work into shorter, manageable units.
2. Then think carefully about your order of presentation.
3. Draw up a list of subheadings and subdivisions, and organize them into a layout that you will use consistently.

Write quickly

Once you have prepared an outline, you can then work towards a first draft of each successive section in your plan by dictating or writing quickly. Leave spaces for the details. You can always look these up later. The priority at this stage is to keep up the flow and momentum of your thoughts. At times when the flow dries up, type the prose into your word processor. At a later date you can refine the text, fill in details, add extra thoughts, correct obvious errors and make sure that your English is appropriate.

Scientific English

Your scientific prose should next undergo a process of evolution and reorganization, with the text being shortened where redundant, expanded, clarified and corrected as necessary with each revision.

1. Make sure that your vocabulary is adequate for, and appropriate to, the subject matter being discussed. This entails being familiar with and understanding the relevant terminology, and making certain that your meaning is clear. Every individual uses different sets of words in different aspects of his or her everyday life. However, in scientific writing, these vocabularies may be inappropriate, or imply a different meaning. Using colloquialisms and stock phrases leads to inaccuracies and misunderstanding, and conveys an impression of lack of care and thought. Select words that best convey your technical meaning, even if a simpler but less accurate word is available. However, subject to the above proviso, use short, clear, familiar words in preference to long unfamiliar ones.
2. Make sure the text is grammatically correct. Sentences should be gener-

ally short, well constructed, and not depart from accepted or appropriate usage.
3. Check that transitions between sentences are smooth and logical. They may mislead the reader if they are too abrupt or misleadingly connected.
4. Make sure the sequence of the argument follows a logical order.
5. Make sure the passage is not written at a level of abstraction inappropriate for the reader.

Re-reading and re-drafting

All drafts, however well planned, demand careful re-reading and correction. After completing the initial version, leave it aside for a few days before you return to it for further work. Your colleagues and supervisor might very helpfully read through and comment on your text. As you approach the final revisions of your text, it is helpful systematically to review the overall content, then the individual paragraphs, sentences and words, as follows.

Content

- Does the text depart from the main point being made in each section?
- Is there padding and irrelevance?
- Could the meaning be made clearer with further examples and illustrations?

Paragraphs

- Does each paragraph form a natural unit?
- Is the transition from one idea or topic illogical or too abrupt?
- Are some topics discussed out of context or left hanging in the air?

Sentences

- Are any sentences too long or involved?
- Are any sentences unclear?
- Are there any pronouns whose antecedents are ambiguous?

Words

- Are there vague, ill-defined words whose meaning is left undefined or unclear?
- Are all terms employed with their accepted scientific meaning?

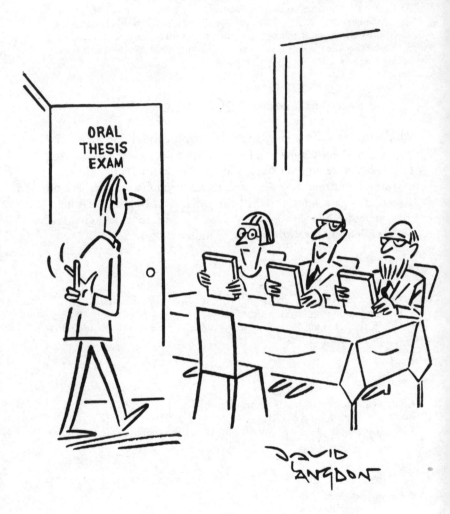

Viva

11

Assembling the thesis

Introduction

Your thesis will contain most or all of the following headings, varying slightly in order, reflecting different university regulations.

- Title page and contents
- Acknowledgements
- Abstract
- Introduction
- Materials and methods
- Results
- Discussion
- Future work and unanswered questions
- Summary
- Glossary and Appendices
- Bibliography or Reference list
- Publications

Title page and contents

Most universities require you or your supervisor to propose a title early in your project. However, you will be able to adjust this at an appropriate stage, once you gather a clear indication of where your research is leading. Take care and advice over your final choice; the title should sum up the essence of your work in a short phrase. The title page should also include your name and address, and any other details that university regulations require.

If you are feeling particularly literate, or want to 'lighten up' a thesis, you might include a quotation. Make sure all quotations are accurate, correctly attributed and are directly relevant to the theme to which they refer.

You should also include a clear contents list at the start of the thesis. Some word processing packages will compile them automatically. (Before final completion, it is prudent to check the contents list to ensure that the titles match those in the book, particularly if the work has been revised since the contents page was originally compiled.) It is also often helpful to have a contents page at the start of each chapter or major section.

Acknowledgements

A separate page should contain a list of acknowledgements, usually set out in paragraphs. If in doubt, choose to include rather than exclude individuals from your acknowledgements.

1. Thank your department head and the laboratory superintendent, at the very least, for access to facilities, and for other help, if this was given.
2. Your supervisor must be thanked.
3. You will wish to thank technicians and laboratory workshops, the computer department, departmental artists, photographer and secretaries who did much of the work in assisting your passage.
4. There will probably be postdoctoral fellows and other colleagues, who will have rendered invaluable aid and advice.
5. Acknowledge all individuals or agencies who lent you equipment.
6. Copyright permission should be included for direct reproductions from published material.
7. You need permission to cite unpublished data or personal communications in your thesis.
8. Be sure to acknowledge your funding body, and any title attached to your scholarship or grant.

Abstract

This is usually controlled by word limit and stipulated format in the university regulations. It is imperative to follow these requirements. The abstract often has to be submitted to regulatory bodies within the university for approval before appointing examiners. It should briefly and succinctly summarize the work performed, and should have a clear paragraphed layout. Remember that it is the first thing that your examiners read when your thesis arrives. It will be referred to repeatedly while it is being examined, again just before your oral examination and, finally, when the examiners compose their report. Much therefore depends on it and the greatest care should be taken in its preparation. It is the shortest part of your thesis, but it is probably the most important!

You should include in your abstract:

1. a few lines stating the overall aims of the work and the early findings that prompted the project;
2. a brief paragraph on the methods and procedures employed, referring particularly to experimental controls;
3. one or more paragraphs outlining the principal experimental findings, in logical sequence (not necessarily described in the chronological order in which they were actually obtained);
4. a summary of the principal conclusions, followed by some reference to their implications.

In the absence of a stipulated word limit, 300 words should usually suffice for this most important section of the thesis.

Introduction

The introduction presents a broad survey of the work of previous investigators in the general field of your thesis and justifies your choice of study. It is often helpful to provide a historical setting: what happened at the beginning, how ideas developed, how new techniques helped, pointing out existing gaps in understanding (to be filled in, of course, by your own work!). The examiners will expect you to demonstrate a deep knowledge and a real understanding of the background to your subject, and the introduction will almost certainly be discussed in your oral examination.

Equally important is a thorough coverage of the set of papers immediately leading up to the work you have done. You must be seen to be familiar with, and to understand, these. You must appreciate both consistencies and contradictions in this earlier work, consider reasons for them, and appreciate their importance. Introducing your own project can then follow naturally. Set out why you chose this particular question and its importance to the general field. Many theses then complete the introduction with some general comments on the experiments, and some indication of the results obtained, to prepare the reader for what is to follow.

If the thesis involves two or more rather separate pieces of work, for example, both experimental and clinical studies of the effects of uraemia on wound healing, then each topic is more easily reviewed separately.

Materials and methods

You should aim to make your methods section:

1. full and explicit: do not skimp on detail by saying 'using the method of Smith and Jones (1987)' without giving a resumé of the method. If necessary, full details could be covered in an appendix.
2. reproducible: there should be enough detail for your experiments to be repeated on a future occasion, without referring to other publications. Diagrams or photographs of your apparatus are useful here.
3. concise: within the above limitations, you should aim to present the method as clearly and concisely as possible.

There are several ways of laying out your methods section.

1. Separate materials and methods sections, for example:

   Materials
   Allopurinol was a gift from the Wellcome Foundation Ltd, Kent, UK. Dulbecco's modification of Eagle's medium and fetal calf serum were purchased from Flow Laboratories Ltd, UK . . .

   Methods
   Palmar fascia was obtained from patients during fasciectomy for Dupuytren's contracture or carpal tunnel release operations for carpal tunnel syndrome . . .

2. A single methods section with details of the materials given throughout the text in brackets, for example:

   1.0 mg of xanthine oxidase (Sigma Ltd, Herts, UK) was added to the incubation media.

   Further details of the materials used may be presented in an appendix.

All statistical methods should be identified. They can be mentioned after describing the relevant method. When several statistical techniques are used, it should be absolutely clear which method was used and where. Very common techniques, such as t-tests, simple χ^2 tests,

Wilcoxon and Mann–Whitney tests, correlation, and linear regression, do not need to be described in detail. Variants of particular methods, such as paired and unpaired t-tests, should be identified unambiguously. More complex methods do require explanation, and precise references should be given for unusual methods. It may be helpful to comment briefly on why a particular method of analysis was used, especially if a more familiar approach was also available. Where appropriate, you should name the computer program or software package used. When doing so, the particular statistical methods employed should still be identified.

Results

Set out your results in a logical order, not necessarily in the chronological sequence in which you actually performed your experiments. Begin with those results which validated the experimental technique, or with the early, simplest and most straightforward results. If appropriate, a careful and systematic description of the data should follow. In general, variables which are important for the validity and subsequent interpretation of statistical analyses should be described in more detail. Liberally use aids to clarify data, such as graphical representation of data, scatter plots or histograms, or summary tables of statistics. Avoid multiple line plots and multiple axes in graphs. It is better to draw such sets of plots separately. You have space in the thesis for this. Follow with the confirmatory experimental results. Leave the more sophisticated or complicated results to the end.

Clarify and emphasize your controls. Deviations from the intended study design should be described. For example, in clinical trials it is important to enumerate withdrawals from treatment allocation, with reasons, if known. In surveys, where the response rate is of fundamental importance, it is valuable to give information on how the non-responders differed from those who took part.

Where there are large amounts of repetitive data, these could be placed in one or more appendices (see later). These might include data such as detailed lists of patients, their age, diagnosis, survival, etc., or long lists of experimental results. If these are incorporated into the main body of your results section, they will disrupt the flow of the thesis. It is quite appropriate to state, for example, 'The results on which Table 10 are based are presented in Appendix 3 on page 139' or 'Clinical details of the 46 patients studied are given in Appendix A on page 141.'

Discussion

The discussion section relates your work to the background of existing knowledge on the subject, and demonstrates how your results have advanced the field. For example, the hypothesis which arose from the research papers you reviewed in your introduction may now have been proven or refuted, the clinical observations of previous workers confirmed and expanded, or your experimental observations may have shed light on that hypothesis.

Many workers begin by summarizing the techniques employed and their validity (if they are new), and the major findings. Although this seems repetitious, it helps you emphasize the major results, so facilitating your arguments to follow. Your examiner also will appreciate a summary at this stage.

This will lead naturally to an immediate interpretation of your findings; outline what your results mean, without extensive details of data analysis, but emphasize comparisons with the controls. You should include enough information and argument to convince your reader of your central message.

You will then wish to relate your results to other findings in a manner that will depend on the nature of your work and the history of the field. For example, your project may have been prompted by earlier findings suggesting an interesting line of study. If so, you need to summarize these earlier findings, what they suggested, and where your findings now lead. Alternatively, you may have sought to resolve apparent (or real) discrepancies between earlier findings. If so, you will want to discuss the extent to which your results resolve the controversy. Finally, you may have entered a little explored area about which hardly anything is known. You will then be presenting a set of novel phenomena, which you should lay out as clearly as possible, before proceeding to more speculative interpretations.

You may wish to conclude with a broader coverage of ideas and hypotheses arising from your results, and their relationship to your surveyed field as a whole.

Future work and unanswered questions

No thesis is ever complete. It has been said that a good thesis will provide its author with enough work to occupy him for the rest of his professional life. The senior author of this present book can vouch for this; he has continued to plod away in clinical and experimental studies based on his thesis on intra-abdominal adhesions for more than a quarter of a century – and still finds more questions which remain unanswered!

Unanswered questions and ideas for future work are sure to come to you. Even if they have not, they are certain to be in the mind of your examiner. Frequent questions asked in oral examinations include 'What further work arising from your thesis might you have in mind?' or 'Did you think of doing a further experiment using X instead of Y?'. It is therefore well worth having a page or two in your thesis which discusses these questions, perhaps four to six of them , and you should devote perhaps one or two paragraphs to each.

Summary

A good summary comes second only in importance to a good abstract in providing an overall review of your thesis. Take each of the main sections of your thesis, Introduction, Materials and methods, Results, Discussion, and Future work, and summarize each of these in a few brief numbered sentences. We have already mentioned how important your abstract is to your examiners. They will also appreciate having a really concise and clear summary to guide them through your thesis.

Glossary

A glossary at the end of the thesis is sometimes used to define terms, abbreviations or unfamiliar concepts.

Appendices

Appendices are often useful for material whose inclusion in the main thesis would disrupt the flow of the text. This might include: epidemiological questionnaires, methods of histological staining, details of statistical tests, clinical details of patients, and computer programs.

Bibliography or Reference list

In the course of your postgraduate work, you will have read papers and reviews whose content now forms the background to your thesis. You need to present all those that you cited in your dissertation in an organized list. A bibliography includes works not referred to directly in the text; a reference list is confined to works referred to in the text. Probably the most convenient way of referring to the literature in your thesis is the Harvard citation system, which gives author and year of publication in the text, and the full reference in the bibliography.

1. In the text, authors' surnames are given in the order in which they appear in the research paper, followed by the date in brackets [e.g. Smith, Martin & Jones (1989)]. In the reference list itself, authors' initials must also be given, and the full reference details.
2. If there are more than three authors, then in the text the first author's name is given followed by '*et al.*' [e.g. 'The validity of the method was investigated by Smith *et al.* (1989) . . .'], but all the authors are named in full in the reference list. [NB This is why while making notes of your references you should keep a record of all the authors; see Chapter 6. Furthermore, some journals ask for the list of authors in full, and it is always easier to delete details than to add them.]
3. If the same authors published more than one paper in the same year, and these works are cited in the text, then the date is suffixed with 'a' or 'b', etc.
4. If the article is a chapter in a book, name the article, and its authors, as well as the title and the editor of the book.
5. Make sure that you use a consistent style of presentation for all the works in the reference list.

Publications

By the time your thesis is bound, you may already have one or more publications in journals, or abstracts in meetings where you presented your results. These should be quoted in the text, and listed in the bibliography. However, it is a good idea to insert the publications themselves into a flap placed inside the back hard cover of your thesis. If you have a paper in press but not yet published, it is still worth having a flap in place. The publication may appear during the delay which often intervenes between thesis submission and your oral examination. You can then bring the reprints with you to your viva, and give them to your examiners.

Successive draftings of the thesis

The first draft of a chapter or section should describe nearly all the experimental details, data and its analyses. References and cross-references to other parts of the thesis can be added later. At this stage your text will therefore be in rough form, but will contain most of the factual material you need to include. There will then be a good deal of moving, adding and deleting of text and checking minor points. Once this initial work is completed, you should read through the first draft to correct obvious mistakes.

In succeeding drafts you will make corrections, add references to the text, adjust the English and vocabulary, and so work towards your final version. Depending on circumstances, it is helpful and instructive for you if your supervisor reads and comments at least on selected chapters as they are being written, preferably at an early stage, to ensure that you are on the right track. However, it is totally unrealistic and inconsiderate to expect your supervisor to drop all his commitments hurriedly to read a belatedly prepared effort given to him at short notice, shortly before a submission deadline. So start writing early to leave yourself and others a lot of time to manoeuvre.

Once all the components of the thesis are assembled, there follows a process of further work, usually pruning, by both yourself and your supervisor. Theses in their early stages are inevitably too long, so do not be too concerned if a great deal of material is subsequently omitted, particularly where there is repetition, or material that is not relevant to the main thrust of the thesis.

Final checklist

The next step is to go through the whole thesis with a fine toothcomb; a stage that may take up to a month! A checklist might include:

Abbreviations. Are they really necessary?
                        Are they explained clearly at the first occurrence?
                        Can the reader find them quickly?
                        Are they consistent?

Format. Check the following for consistency of style and presentation.
- Fonts
- Tables
- Figure legends
- Text headings
- Contents
- References
- Appendices

Numbering. Check that numbering sequences of the following are complete and consistent with references in the text.
- Tables
- Figures
- Text sections

Correctness. Make a final check for accuracy in the following.
- Materials
- Methods
- Statistics
- References
- Figures

Language. Are certain expressions used too frequently?

Tenses. Check that these are correct throughout.

Plurals. e.g. check data/datum, media/medium.

Spelling. Check for correctness and consistency.

Punctuation. Check for accuracy and reliability.

Layout. Does the text start a new page in the correct places?
              Is the page numbering correct?

Units. Make sure that all scientific units (kilograms, litres, etc.) are expressed using the correct abbreviations according to standard reference texts (e.g. *Quantities, Units and Symbols*, the Royal Society of London).

Figures. Make sure that the labelling on these is consistent with the text and legends. Check that you have used the same abbreviations, mathematical symbols, spellings and general style.

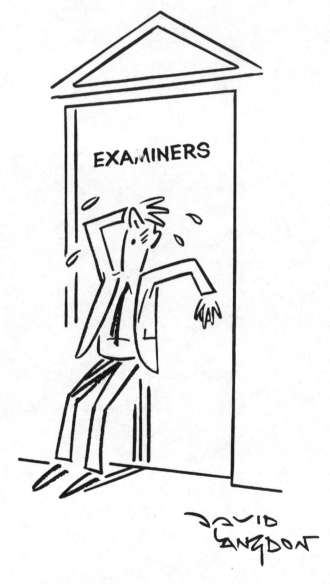

'Phew!'

12

Submitting the thesis

As the time for thesis submission approaches, you will be in a great hurry. You must resist this urge and be fastidious in these final stages, particularly when it comes to printing and binding your thesis. In this way, the consternation of noticing that pages 27–31 are missing, or Figure 4 is upside down, in the final bound version can be avoided!

Number of copies

An important early decision, taken well before you print your photographs and illustrations, is the number of copies of your thesis that you will need. These calculations must take into account how many copies the university requires for submission, and how many it will eventually keep.

Calculating the number of copies of your thesis

	Example
University	3 (2 returned)
Personal	1
Supervisor	1
Departmental head	1
Departmental library	1
Family	1
Close colleagues	2
Total	10

Timing

The printing and binding of your thesis usually takes a much shorter time than you expect; usually a week, but it can even be done over two or three days. Nevertheless, it is important to locate the appropriate photocopier and binder, and find out times and prices, so that you may plan for them.

Printing

Read through your final draft carefully and, if possible, have another person check the draft for errors. Once you have checked and double-checked your thesis text, print it out on a high-quality printer. Even if you are well practised with this printer, there will be unacceptable 'bugs' in the data transmission, and errors in the printing. Plan and be ready for them.

Photocopying

Once you consider that your final draft is as close to perfect as you can make it, take it to the photocopier you have chosen. Choice of photocopying agent will be influenced by the following.

1. Quality: at this stage quality is more important than price. It is of little use to bind beautifully poor-quality photocopies on thin off-white paper!
2. Collation: most good commercial photocopiers will collate the copies for you – a great saving of time.
3. Time: most commercial agents will copy for you overnight. Doing it yourself is a tedious process.
4. Cost: this is the least important consideration at this stage.

Inserting illustrations

1. Stick in your line drawings and re-photocopy the page. Provided the reproduction is of adequate quality, this gives a much more tidy result.
2. Stick in the photographs you do not want to photocopy. Spray-on synthetic adhesives are better than traditional water soluble pastes, which cause pages to wrinkle.
3. Check that each set of manuscripts has the required pages in the correct order.

4. Proof read for the final time. Check that the correct illustrations are attached to each figure legend.

Binding

The binding process will vary from place to place. Have the appropriate number of volumes bound, in a manner acceptable to university regulations.

Submitting

Congratulations! You have now reached the penultimate hurdle. Covet your beautifully prepared volumes. Package and submit them to your university in exactly the fashion they require.

The oral examination

Most candidates for a higher degree by thesis will have an oral examination. Consult your university regulations to find out whether this is obligatory, customary, unusual or never occurs for your particular degree. Some oral examinations include the supervisor, but in most cases you will only encounter two or three examiners.

This is undoubtedly a daunting experience for you; it forms one of the most important days of your professional life and, we can tell you, one that you will never forget! In the days before your examination, you should read through your own copy of the thesis and revise, once again, at least the key references. Arrive early, bring your own copy of your thesis with you and, it should go without saying, turn up neat and tidy. Dirty fingernails can be very off-putting even to the kindest and most considerate examiner.

Usually each examiner in turn asks you questions, and with your replies there may then be subsidiary questions to follow. You are likely to be taken progressively through your thesis. You may first be asked some background questions: where are you working now, what are your future plans, what made you take up this particular field of work? The examiners may then probe your knowledge of the literature (and may well allude to their own work in your field), your findings, your conclusions, where you think you have advanced knowledge in your subject, and finally, where future progress may lie.

Remember one most important thing which should comfort you during your ordeal: you probably know, at this particular moment, just as much, if not more, about your area of work as the examiners do. After all, they did not go through all the references over the previous fortnight, nor have they spent the last year or more devoting all their working time to this particular topic!

The usual procedure is for you to be dismissed at the end of the examination and for the examiners then to make their recommendation to the university. You should hear your official result in a few days. Many examiners, however, will leave you a broad hint of how you fared at the end of your viva.

Further reading

Medawar, P. B. (1981) *Advice to a young scientist*. London: Pan Books.

Calnan, J., Barabas, A. (1972) *Speaking at medical meetings*. London: Heinemann.

Ebel, H. F., Bliefert, C., Russey, W. E. (1987) *The art of scientific writing*. VCH Publications Inc., pp. 29–52.

Bolsky, M. I. (1988) *Better scientific and technical writing*. New Jersey: Prentice Hall.

Hawkins, C., Sorgi, M. (1985) *Research. How to plan, speak and write about it*. Berlin: Springer Verlag.

Booth, V. (1985) *Communicating in science: writing and speaking*. Cambridge University Press.

Appendix:
Information for research students
wishing to study overseas

International

International handbook of universities and other institutions of higher education. Guide to universities in 108 other countries outside the Commonwealth, USA, Ireland and South Africa. Edited by H. M. R. Keyes and D. J. Aitken. De Gruyter: Hawthorn, NY.

World list of universities. Guide to 6000 universities in 150 countries. De Gruyter: Hawthorn, NY.

Study abroad. Lists scholarships, assistantships, travel grants, international courses in all fields of study, offered, sponsored or administered by more than 70 international organizations. UNESCO Press: Paris.

The grants register. Lists grants, scholarships, special awards, etc., for anyone requiring further professional or occupational training. Edited by Roland Turner. MacMillan Press: London.

The Commonwealth

Commonwealth universities yearbook. The standard guide to the courses, organization, staff and activities of about 500 university institutions of good standing in 29 countries or regions of the Commonwealth. Published annually by the Association of Commonwealth Universities, John Foster House, 36 Gordon Square, London, England WC1H 0PF.

Scholarships guide for Commonwealth postgraduate students. Published every two years by the Association of Commonwealth Universities, John Foster House, 36 Gordon Square, London, England WC1H 0PF.

Awards for Commonwealth university staff. Fellowships, visiting professorships, grants, etc. open to university staff in a commonwealth country wishing to study in another country. Published every two years by the Association of Commonwealth Universities, 36 Gordon Square, London, England WC1H 0PF.

Awards for postgraduate study overseas. Handbook of grants 1 & 2. (ed. M. Brown.) Handy, concise lists of recurring scholarships and grants for postgraduates, post doctorates and academics studying in Australia. For Australians and citizens of other countries. Available from the Graduate Careers Council of Australia, PO Box 28, Parkville, Victoria 3052, Australia or scholarships office of the local University. Free of charge.

Graduate study at universities in Britain. A short student information paper including the names of guides to advanced study or research in separate subjects. Association of Commonwealth Universities, 36 Gordon Square, London, WC1H 0PF. (Stamped addressed envelope or two International Reply coupons required.)

British universities guide to graduate study. Published every two years by the Association of Commonwealth Universities, 36 Gordon Square, London WC1H 0PF.

Higher Education in the United Kingdom. Published every two years by the Association of Commonwealth Universities, 36 Gordon Square, London WC1H 0PF.

Research strengths of universities in the developing countries of the Commonwealth. A register of what universities in the developing countries can offer in the way of research facilities to staff and graduate students. Published by the Association of Commonwealth Universities, 36 Gordon Square, London, England WC1H 0PF.

Postgraduate study at universities in Britain. A short informational paper containing the names of guides to advanced study or research in separate subjects. Association of Commonwealth Universities, 36 Gordon Square, London, England WC1H 0PF.

United States of America

American universities and colleges. The standard guide to universities and colleges in the US. Edited by W. Todd Furniss. American Council of Education, 1 Dupont Circle, Washington DC 20036, USA.

A selected list of fellowship opportunities and aids to advanced education for United States citizens and foreign nationals. The Publications Office, National Science Foundation, 1800 G Street, NW, Washington DC 20550, USA.

Graduate programs and admissions manual. Information on postgraduate programmes in the USA. Includes details on the admissions processes, financial aid, test requirements, student–staff ratios and full addresses of all listed institutions. Education Testing Service, Princeton, NJ 08541, USA.

Entering Higher Education in the United States: a guide for students from other countries. New York, College Board, Publications Orders, Box 2815, Princeton, NJ 08541, USA.

Financial planning for study in the United States. New York, College Board, Publications Orders, Box 2815, Princeton, NJ 08541, USA.

The college handbook. Describes more than 2800 US colleges and universities with basic information about each one. New York, College Board, Publications Orders, Box 2815, Princeton, NJ 08541, USA.

Australian–American Postgraduate Foundation, PO Box 1559, Canberra City, ACT 2601, Australia. This organization provides information on study in the US. They stress that financial aid for US universities and colleges, usually in the form of assistantships and tuition waivers, is difficult to get. Information regarding financial aid can only be obtained from the institutions themselves by writing to the appropriate department head of the financial aids office of the individual institution.

Index